Routledge Revivals

The Doctor's Job

Originally published in 1946, *The Doctor's Job* is an account of changes in medicine over the decades, focusing on the rapid expansion of medical science and the development of specialties. Carl Binger, a distinguished psychiatrist and physician and pioneer in psychosomatic medicine, reflects on the ethical, emotional, and intellectual challenges faced by doctors at the time and the evolving role of medicine in society. Today it can be read in its historical context.

This book is a re-issue originally published in 1946. The language used is a reflection of its era and no offence is meant by the Publishers to any reader by this re-publication.

The Doctor's Job

Carl Binger

Routledge
Taylor & Francis Group
Routledge Revivals

First published in Great Britain in 1946
by George Allen & Unwin Ltd

This edition first published in 2026 by Routledge
4 Park Square, Milton Park, Abingdon, Oxon, OX14 4RN

and by Routledge
605 Third Avenue, New York, NY 10158

Routledge is an imprint of the Taylor & Francis Group, an informa business

Publisher's Note
The publisher has gone to great lengths to ensure the quality of this reprint but points out that some imperfections in the original copies may be apparent.

Disclaimer
The publisher has made every effort to trace copyright holders and welcomes correspondence from those they have been unable to contact.

ISBN: 978-1-041-19396-8 (hbk)
ISBN: 978-1-003-71158-2 (ebk)
ISBN: 978-1-041-19400-2 (pbk)

Book DOI 10.4324/9781003711582

THE DOCTOR'S JOB

by

CARL BINGER
M.D.

. . . any man's *death*
diminishes *me*, because
I am involved in
Mankinde

JOHN DONNE, *Devotions*

London
GEORGE ALLEN & UNWIN LTD

First published in Great Britain
in 1946

PRINTED IN GREAT BRITAIN BY
HENDERSON AND SPALDING, LONDON, W.1

TO

DAVID LINN EDSALL

Dean Emeritus of the Harvard Medical School

TEACHER AND FRIEND

THE OATH OF HIPPOCRATES

I SWEAR BY APOLLO PHYSICIAN, BY ASCLEPIUS, BY HEALTH, BY PANACEA AND BY ALL THE GODS AND GODDESSES, MAKING THEM MY WITNESSES, THAT I WILL CARRY OUT, ACCORDING TO MY ABILITY AND JUDGMENT, THIS OATH AND THIS INDENTURE. TO HOLD MY TEACHER IN THIS ART EQUAL TO MY OWN PARENTS; TO MAKE HIM PARTNER IN MY LIVELIHOOD; WHEN HE IS IN NEED OF MONEY TO SHARE MINE WITH HIM; TO CONSIDER HIS FAMILY AS MY OWN BROTHERS, AND TO TEACH THEM THIS ART, IF THEY WANT TO LEARN IT, WITHOUT FEE OR INDENTURE; TO IMPART PRECEPT, ORAL INSTRUCTION, AND ALL OTHER INSTRUCTION TO MY OWN SONS, THE SONS OF MY TEACHER, AND TO INDENTURED PUPILS WHO HAVE TAKEN THE PHYSICIAN'S OATH, BUT TO NOBODY ELSE. I WILL USE TREATMENT TO HELP THE SICK ACCORDING TO MY ABILITY AND JUDGMENT, BUT NEVER WITH A VIEW TO INJURY AND WRONGDOING. NEITHER WILL I ADMINISTER A POISON TO ANYBODY WHEN ASKED TO DO SO, NOR WILL I SUGGEST SUCH A COURSE. SIMILARLY I WILL NOT GIVE TO A WOMAN A PESSARY TO CAUSE ABORTION. BUT I WILL KEEP PURE AND HOLY BOTH MY LIFE AND MY ART. I WILL NOT USE THE KNIFE, NOT EVEN, VERILY, ON SUFFERERS FROM STONE, BUT I WILL GIVE PLACE TO SUCH AS ARE CRAFTSMEN THEREIN. INTO WHATSOEVER HOUSES I ENTER, I WILL ENTER TO HELP THE SICK, AND I WILL ABSTAIN FROM ALL INTENTIONAL WRONGDOING AND HARM, ESPECIALLY FROM ABUSING THE BODIES OF MAN OR WOMAN, BOND OR FREE. AND WHATSOEVER I SHALL SEE OR HEAR IN THE COURSE OF MY PROFESSION, AS WELL AS OUTSIDE MY PROFESSION IN MY INTERCOURSE WITH MEN, IF IT BE WHAT SHOULD NOT BE PUBLISHED ABROAD, I WILL NEVER DIVULGE, HOLDING SUCH THINGS TO BE HOLY SECRETS. NOW IF I CARRY OUT THIS OATH, AND BREAK IT NOT, MAY I GAIN FOR EVER REPUTATION AMONG ALL MEN FOR MY LIFE AND FOR MY ART; BUT IF I TRANSGRESS IT AND FORSWEAR MYSELF, MAY THE OPPOSITE BEFALL ME.

Contents

Foreword

THIS book was begun at Little Compton, Rhode Island, while I was lying on my back on the beach or sitting under some ancient elms. Most of it, however, was written in the midst of a busy life in New York.

I have tried to give an account of some of the changes that have taken place in medicine in the last few decades—many of them within my personal experience, most within the experience of my teachers. The rapid expansion of medical science, the disappearance of the encyclopedic wise man who knew all there was to know, the development of specialties and of specialists have been discussed. How this scientific growth brought its great benefits, but also how the sick man himself became the forgotten man in the face of the battery of tests to which he was exposed, have been made evident. The importance of the relationship of physician and patient has been emphasized, not as a sentimental one but as containing within it the so-called *transference* situation which, by mechanisms now better understood, possesses stupendous powers for good and ill. I have dealt with psychoanalysis and its revolutionary influence both in psychiatry and in medicine and have sketched the outlines of psychosomatic medicine, dealing, as this does, with the subtle interplay of mind and body. The problem of "cure" has been considered and stock has been taken of recent achievements and future tasks.

With the brilliantly won battle against infant mortality and early death from infection came the lengthening of the average life span and a corresponding increase in the number of sufferers from the chronic diseases of middle and late life. These diseases raise many problems of a social and economic nature—among others, that of convalescent care. In many respects the relative predominance of such chronic diseases has changed the doctor's job. All this has led naturally to a consideration of the prevention of illness—perhaps the physician's most important and challenging task—and to a discussion of medicine as it is practiced in office, hospital and outpatient department. The perplexing issues springing from increased costs of medical care have been weighed. No doctrinaire schemes for salvation have been offered up, but instead I have tried to emphasize what constitutes good medical care. In the final chapter I have outlined the silhouette of that ancient oak—our medical family tree—whose roots are in prehistory and whose branches spread out over life.

A number of my friends, medical and lay, have let me read parts of the manuscript to them and have made helpful comments. My classmate and colleague, Dr. Henry Alden Bunker, listened to it chapter by chapter and brought to it the illumination of his scholarly mind. Dr. Thomas A. C. Rennie read the manuscript and benefited it by his taste and by the breadth of his experience. Dr. Horace Gray pointed up the bricks of this edifice with a skillful and delicate hand.

I wish also to acknowledge my warm gratitude to the skipper and cook of the Sloop *Fulmar*, Dr. and Mrs. Stanley Cobb. Our annual cruises, interrupted only by the restrictions of war, were the setting for much pleasant talk which has helped to clarify my thoughts. As Marcel Proust has it, we are able to get lucidity only from those individuals whose ideas are in the same state of confusion as our own.

My thanks go to Warder Norton for his encouragement and assistance, to my friend Francis W. Roudebush for executing the jacket lettering, to my secretary Mrs. Charlotte Lieman for her painstaking deciphering and typing of manuscript, and to my wife for her help in all the activities, overt and submerged, that go into the making of a book.

C. B.

Introduction

NO ONE can write about his profession—or perhaps about anything else—without revealing himself. Such self-revelation will amount to an autobiography. A man's occupation is, to be sure, a kind of self-revelation. However circumstantial the causes for following a profession or doing a job in this world, there lie behind the purely superficial reasons certain subjective ones which find their expression in our occupations. These need not always be the same. Men study medicine for divers reasons: some to make scientific discoveries, others to help their fellow men, and still others to experience "life" in its manifold aspects. Any one of these should suffice as an explanation. The deeper causes are the concern of the individual himself, for the final test of a man's work is not his underlying impulses but what he does with them, and whether they are happily converted into socially useful and creative ends, rather than into destructive ones.

My own approach to medicine came early in life, at about the age of nine. I had a dog named Chief, a smooth-haired fox terrier, not a very elegant animal in retrospect. He often strayed from home and after thirteen years he ran away, never to return. He was constantly in trouble. He would come back bedraggled, mangy and bitten. Once he jumped through a glass windowpane. I used to bathe his wounds and bandage him and wait hopefully while God cured him. I had my appendix out at about the same time. The operation was done at home and all the preparations were visible to my inquiring eyes. I had a beautiful nurse who seemed very cool and majestic. All of these circumstances undoubtedly led me in the direction of medicine, but in addition certain inner forces impelled me to tackle the doctor's job.

Many doctors, reflecting on their careers, may discover that therapeutic interest, or a desire to heal, has governed their work. The truly great minds in medicine have often been free from this. Perhaps nothing of the sort activated a Harvey, a Claude Bernard or a Freud. Still, for the man who practices medicine and deals with sick people, a desire to heal cannot be a disadvantage unless he allows it to blind him to the nature of the problems with which he deals or makes him indulge in hit or miss empirical short cuts. And so the wish to heal has taken me to many places, as it has other physicians—into hospital wards, laboratories, tenements and marble halls, into army camps, into the wild and barren uplands of eastern Macedonia, the high Andes of Peru and into the dark recesses of the human spirit where there is both squalor and grandeur. No one in medicine is wise enough to comprehend what he daily beholds. Nothing a man has of scientific acumen, personal integrity and human understanding is too much to bring to this job. And only seldom will the results achieved be commensurate with the effort, the responsibility and the long period of training.

The public is so often impatient with us physicians. As their own enlightenment has increased so our prestige has waned. Do they really want to be humbugged? Is the need for magic so great in them and its effects so potent that our patients will always turn away to the cultist and the quack for relief from suffering? Can the man of medicine unmask himself and cease his incantations and still be the healer of the sick? I believe he can, but not without a critical and conscious awareness of what he is doing and of what he represents to his patients. I intend to discuss some of these problems: the old one of the doctor-patient relationship, the choice of the physician, the much derided problem of medical ethics, the matter of fees, socialized medicine, the passing of the family doctor, the need and province of the specialist, the gradual return of medicine from its purely technical concerns to its more humane and psychiatric beginnings and, lastly, psychosomatic medicine, or that newly hatched but venerable baby which deals with the relationships of mind and body. Much has been written on these subjects, more will be. I am setting down these thoughts now because I feel the need of doing so.

CHAPTER I

Background and Changes

TIME was, and not so long ago, when the family doctor delivered babies and supervised their nursing, their weaning and their teething, when he vaccinated them and saw them through their measles and chicken pox and whooping cough. He told the boy about the facts of life and treated the girl for her menstrual cramps. He advised about diet and rest, gave spring tonics, clipped tonsils, set a broken arm, reassured father who couldn't sleep because of business worries, pulled mother through a case of typhoid or double pneumonia, reprimanded the cook who was found, on her day out, to have a dozen empty whisky bottles in her clothes closet, gave advice about the young man's choice of college and profession, comforted grandma, who was losing her memory and becoming more and more irritable, and closed grandpa's eyes in his final sleep. He went on his endless, mysterious and incessant rounds leaving in his wake a faint odor of carbolic with which he disinfected his beard. This heroic figure is gone from our midst. He survives only in a few remaining rural communities where, like the anachronistic hitching post, he stands as a memorial to our simpler and more rugged past. Nor can all our nostalgic longings wish him back into existence. Who killed Cock Robin? What combination of circumstances banished him?

The superficial causes for his disappearance are not far to seek. To attend to the rather simple medical needs of a family such as I have just described would today require the services not of one man but probably of six: an obstetrician, a pediatrician, a nose and throat doctor, a surgeon, a psychiatrist and an internist. Our question is, what forces or circumstances brought these new characters onto the medical stage and led to the exit of the old-fashioned general practitioner? To dig to the roots of this problem or to see it as a part only of a far larger social evolution would require the knowledge of an expert sociologist. Certainly the industrial revolution, the great concentration of populations in urban centers, the loosening of home and community ties must all have had their share of influence. But as one looks at the problem more immediately the outstanding fact is that the new members of the caste we call specialists have acquired, each in his own field, a technical knowledge and often a manual skill that no one man can master. A modern tonsillectomy is as different from an old-fashioned tonsil-clipping procedure as an oil-burning, turbine-engined liner is from a Mississippi side-wheeler. And the modern treatment of pneumonia requires a knowledge of bacteriology, physiology and chemotherapy that did not exist a decade ago.

Thus the first cause for the disappearance of the general practitioner in the old sense of the term is to be found in the vast expansion of medical science which has resulted from the patient labors of research workers.

Other causes operated, too. With the growth of our population and its increased density in urban centers a greater number of graduates in medicine began to compete with each other. It became necessary for survival to know something that the other man did not, or at least to know it better. And so the more enterprising physicians began to cross the Atlantic for postgraduate study, after having spent several struggling years in general practice. Also, it was in the gentleman's tradition to travel and study and many were driven at great sacrifice by a passion for learning. Some went to Germany where medicine was still in its golden age, as yet unspoiled by authoritarianism—to Berlin and Munich and Heidelberg and Würzburg and Leipzig for pathology and bacteriology, for physiology and internal medicine—and, of course, to Vienna. Some went to Dublin to study midwifery at the famous Rotunda. Some went to Edinburgh and Paris for surgery—and to Paris also they traveled for studies with Charcot in neurology at the Salpêtrière and with Janet in psychiatry.

A stream of pioneers they were—gifted men, many of them, who returned with their lamps of learning burnished to set up small foci of radiating light from which they illuminated others. Not a few became professors in our medical schools. And some became the great consultants and diagnosticians of the past, our elder Janeways, our Austin Flints, our Oslers—great names and great personalities behind whose brows lay the accumulated knowledge, experience and wisdom of medical generations. Gone are these, too, these Supreme Court justices of medicine, to be replaced by our particular brand of wise man—ready witted, practical, traveling light, less cultivated, a little brittle and jejune but competent, industrious and sometimes inspired. Medicine has entered the loose-leaf age where knowledge is so vast and so changing that it can no longer be bound between cardboards and certainly not lodged within the confines of a single cranium And with its confession of ignorance it has lost some of its power and much of its prestige.

And then came the second migration. By scores, young and middle-aged men went to Germany and to Vienna to study some specialty. After one, two or three years they came home with broadened horizons, a taste for good food and good drink and often for good music. They set themselves up as specialists. They "did" skin or they "did" eye, ear, nose and throat or surgery or obstetrics and gynecology. It took courage and foresight to make this break. Some of them continued with a certain amount of general practice to eke out a slender income. The more adventurous braved it out, burned their bridges to wait for private patients. They busied themselves in hospital wards and dispensaries. Then their day arrived. They were able to charge larger fees and to approach their work with perhaps a little more sense of leisure and thoughtfulness. And the ones who stayed at home to do the yeoman's job were the general practitioners who labored and sweated at two or three dollars a visit—up at night and out early in the morning, rich and poor alike, hospital work, civic responsibilities and striving always to keep up with the ever growing mass of literature, much of which they could not even remotely understand. They lacked the training in the fundamental sciences of chemistry, physics and biology, and therefore much of the work in bacteriology, pathology and physiology was unintelligible to them. They became "just general practitioners," engulfed by the changing tides of events.

By the time I graduated in medicine in 1914 the *Drang nach Osten* had somewhat subsided. Men began to specialize earlier. In many of our better teaching hospitals the internships were divided between medicine and surgery. There was opportunity for working in the various outpatient departments and for choosing between such subjects as neurology and skin disease, genitourinary surgery and gynecology. There was already a staff of experts to instruct the young. And another subtle change was going on. Some of the more gifted and ambitious interns were invited by the chiefs of service to stay on as resident physicians. At the time I was an intern these men acted in an advisory capacity when their advice was sought, but they did not run the service as they so often do now. Nor did they rob the senior intern of that rapture of being the hub of his universe, on whose young shoulders all responsibility lay. My old friend and teacher the late John J. Abel, professor of pharmacology at the Johns Hopkins Medical School, who had many honors heaped upon him in his distinguished and useful life, used to say that on the day he got his Ph.D. degree he reached a pinnacle of professional success from which he ever thereafter receded. The same was true of the senior internship. Suddenly, though after what seemed a long vigil, you had won your spurs. The present system, however, of putting older and more experienced residents in charge of the services is undoubtedly better for the ward patients. Usually the residents busied themselves with some form of research problem. I remember when I was an intern that one of our residents had just returned from England where he had learned the new technique of electrocardiography—now become a routine form of examination. Another spent hours alone in a modest and ill-equipped laboratory working with many-colored solutions, studying the reactions of the human body and trying to impart to us the meaning of the hydrogen ion and of acid-base equilibria. He is now a professor of medicine in one of our leading schools who, happily, sees the problems of medicine in the round. Devoted men these were and others like them, men who foreswore marriage and money and gave themselves to their tasks.

Other changes were at work. Fourth-year medical students began to "walk the wards" as clinical clerks. This gave them their first direct contact with the sickbed which heretofore had been pretty much confined to the distant and detached spectacle of amphitheater demonstrations. And at faculty meetings the clinical men and the laboratory men were no longer arrayed in hostile groups on either side of a long table, glowering at each other and bargaining for the souls of the medical students, while a distracted dean or university president tried to pour oil on troubled waters.

When I was a student a shift in emphasis had already occurred. The autopsy room, where so many of our predecessors had spent hours of concentrated labor, was giving way to the physiological laboratory, and, correspondingly, in the clinic a brilliant and correct diagnosis (sometimes, to be sure, only corroborated at post-mortem examination) was no longer the supreme intellectual achievement. Insight and understanding of mechanisms and processes became increasingly important. The dynamic view was ascendant. No longer were anatomists content with describing bones, muscles and nerves, or pathologists with describing the gross and microscopic appearance of tissues. Experiment entered all these domains as it did the domain of medicine and surgery, and before long it became difficult to tell from the nature of the problem and the equipment in use what department you were in. The ancient, fixed, traditional academic borders were breaking down.

But I have anticipated my story. In 1910 an event occurred in American medicine that proved to be both shattering and creative. A bomb burst in the smug and stuffy air. Mr. Abraham Flexner exploded it. Under the auspices of the Carnegie Foundation for the Advancement of Teaching, he investigated all the medical schools in the country and then published a painstaking, detailed and critical description of each. The report disclosed a shocking situation in many: low standards for admission, poor equipment, inadequate clinical facilities and didactic instruction, both antiquated and routine. Many of the schools were proprietary ones conducted by a small group of practitioners for their own advantage, and many were mere diploma mills. This was no muckraking enterprise. The effect was electrifying. It was the spark for a great movement of reform.

Few public exposures, I suspect, have borne fruit so quickly. Nothing in my medical lifetime has had a more profound effect on medical education in this country. If the great foundations had done nothing else with their millions this alone would have been worthwhile, for a standard was raised in medicine to which the wise and honest could repair.

Long before these events—so the story goes—when President Eliot proposed giving written examinations to medical students, Dr. Henry Jacob Bigelow objected on the grounds that too many of them were illiterate. Bigelow was the brilliant professor of surgery who, with Oliver Wendell Holmes, Sr., had most weight in the Harvard medical faculty of the sixties and seventies and who for nearly forty years was the dominating figure in New England surgery. To President Eliot is due the credit for the first great reform in the system of medical education in this country. In his report for 1871–72 he wrote: "It would be difficult to overstate the importance of the effort which this single school is making. . . . The ignorance and general incompetency of the average graduate of American medical schools, at the time when he receives the degree which turns him loose upon the community, is something horrible to contemplate, considering the nature of a physician's functions and responsibilities. . . ."

But his reforms were hard won in the face of selfishness and cynicism on the part of his own faculty and ignorance on the part of the public. Bigelow opposed him with uncompromising and strenuous obstinacy. Referring to that venerable body, the Harvard Corporation, Dr. Bigelow expostulated: "Who are the Corporation? Does Mr. Lowell know anything about medical education? Or the Rev. Dr. Putnam? . . . Why, Mr. Crowninshield carries a horse chestnut in his pocket to keep off rheumatism! Is the new medical education to be best directed by a man who carries horse chestnuts in his pocket to cure rheumatism?"

With the second reform movement initiated by the Flexner report the requirements for admission to medical schools were raised, though I am constantly amazed at the narrow margin of general culture that bounds the horizons of even some of our cleverest contemporary medical students. Within the decade after 1910, the experiment started at the Johns Hopkins Medical School for graduate instruction on a high academic level became standard for the whole country, and the stiffened requirements of the state licensing boards helped to improve the quality of medical practice.

Shortly after the Flexner report, and partly as a consequence of it, came the establishment of full-time chairs of medicine whose occupants for the first time in this country devoted themselves wholly to teaching and research and not to private practice. Other reforms followed. Tedious and soporific hours of didactic lectures gave way to conferences with tutors. Research and investigation were encouraged in specially gifted students. The comprehensive examination was introduced which not only tested a student's knowledge of facts but his ability to marshal them and correlate them. Throughout, the tendency has been toward a better grounding in the fundamental sciences, an awakened interest in chemical and physiological body processes, and a view of medicine not as a corpus of traditional teaching but as an expanding, ever changing discipline built on observation and experiment.

With developments in medical education came also enormous endowments for medical research, the founding of institutes, and emphasis on the ability to investigate as a prerequisite for appointment to a professorship in medicine. Much of a purely casuistic nature was ground out in the hope of furthering the careers of some of the dull but faithful. But work of a high order, both theoretically and from a practical point of view, has flowed pretty steadily from this wellspring of activity. Examples of such far-reaching discoveries are the insulin treatment of diabetes, the use of liver extract and its chemical derivatives in the treatment of pernicious anemia, the whole complicated and modern field of vitamin research and, of course, the miracle of the so-called sulfa drugs. Thanks to the excellent publicity our better newspapers have given to medical discoveries of recent years, the lay public has managed to keep pretty well abreast of them. But they are often unaware of the prehistory of these discoveries, the cost in time and equipment, the gradual development and evolution of thought until the occasion is instant for them, and the changes in practice that follow in their wake.

Whereas the physician began as a single, self-sufficient organism, he has gone through a kind of metamorphosis. What is called in cellular biology a process of maturation has taken place, a growth by division and multiplication, a differentiation, as in a biological organism, resulting in the development of specialized sense organs (the X-ray for example) and specialized skills. What these specialties are I shall discuss in the next chapter, and what their effects have been on sick human beings in later ones.

Major Barbara's father said to her: "You have learnt something. That always feels at first as if you had lost something."

CHAPTER II

Specialties and Specialists

WHEN my mother was young she was cared for medically by a benign old uncle known in her family as Uncle Doctor. He had a Santa Claus beard and wore, in winter, a dark-blue overcoat of broadcloth with a fur collar and a truncated black hat of the Churchill type. He played chess and loved chamber music. I saw him only a few times—once in front of our own house, where his horse had slipped on the ice and fallen. "Uncle Doctor" sat patiently on the animal's head thumbing through some notes while his coachman went off for a bucket of ashes. When my mother was an old woman and pretty worldly wise she once asked me a medical question. I told her I did not know the answer. She looked at me with amazement and incredulity. In the span of her lifetime, and even in mine, the change had occurred from the omniscient Santa Claus to the well-trained, ignorant specialist.

The Directory of The American Medical Association lists twenty-six specialties. Here they are, with a few interpretive remarks:

Allergy—deals with such conditions as hay fever, asthma and sensitiveness to various foods.

Anesthesiology—administration of anesthetics; some by inhalation; others by injection.

Bacteriology—the study, usually for diagnostic purposes, of infectious agents in the blood and in the bodily excretions. This includes also the preparation of vaccines and other forms of immunization.

Cardiovascular Disease—diseases of the heart and blood vessels.

Clinical Pathology—concerns itself with the examination of the blood and of secretions and excretions by chemical and microscopic methods.

Dermatology—diseases of the skin. This specialty usually includes syphilology as well.

Gastroenterology—diseases of the stomach and intestines.

Gynecology—diseases of the female generative organs.

Industrial Medicine—concerns itself chiefly with protection against occupational hazards such as exposure to poisoning by lead or other chemicals.

Internal Medicine—is discussed in this chapter.

Neurology—deals with disorders of the central or peripheral nervous system, that is, the brain, spinal cord and nerves. It may or may not be combined with the practice of psychiatry.

Neurosurgery—the surgery of the brain, spinal cord and nerves.

Obstetrics—or midwifery.

Ophthalmology—diseases of the eye. An ophthalmologist is sometimes called an oculist. An optician is a maker of or dealer in optical instruments who may, when licensed, fit glasses, but he is not equipped by training to examine or treat the eyes.

Orthopedic Surgery—the surgery of bones and joints and the correction of deformities. The word orthopedic is derived from the Greek ὄρθος (straight) and παῖς (child). Although orthopedists frequently aim to correct deformities of the feet, the Latin *pes* (foot) does not contribute to their name.

Otology, Laryngology, Rhinology—this is the medical term for the specialty that treats diseases of the ear, throat and nose.

Pathology—study of abnormal tissues. It is the pathologist who is often called upon to decide whether a tumor removed at operation is benign or malignant.

Pediatrics—diseases of infancy and childhood.

Plastic Surgery—corrective and cosmetic surgery.

Psychiatry—deals with disturbances of the mental and emotional life. Psychiatrists should be distinguished from psychologists who are, as a rule, not doctors of medicine but Ph.D.'s, and whose concern is with experimental studies of mental phenomena and with the administration of certain tests for intelligence, for aptitudes and for inventory of the personality.

Proctology—diseases of the rectum.

Public Health—is concerned mostly with sanitation and the prevention and control of epidemic diseases.

Roentgenology, Radiology—X-ray diagnosis and treatment.

Surgery—usually refers to major surgical operations on the abdomen and chest, but includes also many other fields as, for example, operations on the thyroid gland and the treatment of wounds and fractures.

Tuberculosis—usually of the lungs but may also involve the skin, bones and other organs.

Urology—a branch of surgery that is concerned with disorders of the genital organs, kidneys and bladder—sometimes called genitourinary diseases.

This is the officially recognized list of specialties. For many of them there are qualifying examinations and diplomas issued by certifying boards.

There is also, of course, a category called "general practice" but it will be appreciated from what has gone before that general practice is no longer the omnibus it once was. It is now closer to that specialty called "internal medicine" on which I shall comment presently. In some communities general practice is still combined with such work as minor surgery and obstetrics, but this is naturally truer in localities where there are fewer doctors and where a specialist could not make a living.

As we look over the imposing galaxy of specialties they group themselves naturally into discrete constellations. Around the central sun of general surgery, for example, revolve the separate planets of neurosurgery, oral surgery, orthopedic surgery, urology, anesthesiology. Ophthalmology, or the study of the diseases of the eye, has pretty much separated itself from diseases of the ear, nose and throat. Bronchoscopy is closely related to treatment of diseases of the lungs and the upper respiratory tract. But the technique of instrumentation is so delicate and the interpretation of the picture the operator sees when he squints into a bronchus so confusing that only a master who wields the instrument constantly could wield it at all.

Other particularized and dangerous techniques such as deep X-ray therapy no one but an expert should attempt. But even where manual skill and familiarity with apparatus are not the prime consideration, proficiency can often be assured only by constantly repeated experience.

The early diagnosis of pulmonary tuberculosis is a case in point. Everyone knows that prompt discovery of the lesion in the lung is of utmost importance in preventing its spread and arresting the disease. Subsequent cure depends not only on a strict regime of rest but often on such procedures as artificial pneumothorax, or collapsing the diseased lung by introducing air through a hollow needle inserted through the chest wall into the pleural sac, i.e., into the space that lies between the inside of the chest wall and the lung. All this is naturally far more expertly and safely done by a man constantly in contact with tuberculosis than by a general practitioner or internist who, because of the nature of his practice, encounters sufferers from this malady only occasionally. Paderewski is said to have remarked that when he missed one day of practice he was himself aware of a difference in his performance and when he missed two days his public noticed it.

What was once a simple matter of pouring some ether from a can into a gauze mask and clapping it over a patient's nose and mouth has become an elaborate ceremonial. When I was an intern we used this method and would let the patient up for air when he turned blue. How different now the battery of cylinders and valves with measured flow of gas and mixtures to choose from and control! The patient's color and blood pressure and pulse rate are constantly observed. A skillful anesthetist will keep his patient not only insensible to pain but in a satisfactory state of muscular relaxation and will allow him to "come out" as the operation nears its close. Sometimes he administers carbon dioxide in such concentrations as to stimulate deep breathing for the purpose of washing out the remaining ether vapor from the blood stream. And there are, of course, many volatile anesthetics other than ether, and still other nonvolatile ones given by rectum, or into a vein or intraspinally. This field, too, has become pretty much the province of the expert.

The administration of oxygen, once a futile, eleventh-hour gesture designed to comfort the relatives of the moribund patient, has become a useful and precisely controlled procedure. Formerly a glass funnel was held over the patient's nose and the room air was wastefully inundated with oxygen—not, however, sufficient either to raise its concentration in the atmosphere or to alter the oxygen content of the air in the lungs and thus of the arterial blood. Now, by the use of a nasal catheter or by placing the patient in a specially designed leakproof tent or chamber, a known and indicated dose of oxygen can be supplied and the effect estimated by analyzing the arterial blood for its oxygen content. If given early enough, before the central nervous system has suffered permanent damage from want of oxygen, the modern methods can often prolong life until some specific remedy or natural recuperative powers have become effective.

The modern treatment for syphilis of the central nervous system is no longer an endless series of mercury inunctions with little hope for improvement at the end of them. It has become a combination of procedures: artificial fever deliberately induced by giving the patient injections of blood from an individual suffering from malaria, or by exposing him to external heat from incandescent lamps, or generating heat within his tissues by short, radiolike waves—this combined with specific drugs of a complicated and poisonous nature. And the end result, while perhaps not all that could be desired, is a great step forward.

Perhaps I have said enough to make my point clear. I shall not need to enlarge further on the particular nature of the specialties, much of which must be familiar to the reader. I have already referred to the field known as internal medicine. This is a term in common use in professional circles, but it has never been taken up by the lay public. I doubt whether the so-called man on the street would know what an internist is. He might possibly know that a pediatrician takes care of sick children, if indeed he didn't confuse him with a podiatrist—a parlor name for a chiropodist.

Internal medicine derives from the German *Innere Medizin*, an academic conception that grew up in the famous university clinics. It is not primarily concerned with the entrails of the body but rather with the inwardness of medicine—the core after the appendages have been lopped off. It concerns itself with diseases involving organs and organ systems. The province of internal medicine includes acute infectious diseases such as pneumonia or typhoid or rheumatic fever; disturbances of body chemistry such as diabetes or gout or nephritis (kidney disease), of the glands of internal secretion such as disorders of the thyroid gland; degenerative diseases associated with aging, such as arthritis, arteriosclerosis or hardening of the arteries, high blood pressure and various forms of heart disease; also various disturbances of the digestive and respiratory systems such as stomach ulcer, colitis, asthma. A competent internist should be reasonably at home in all of these fields. He should be familiar with many diagnostic procedures and, above all, he should know what experts to call upon when his own knowledge or technical skill is inadequate to the problem at hand. He will have frequent recourse to the X-ray apparatus, the electrocardiograph, the serological laboratory, where such tests as the Wassermann reaction for syphilis are carried out. He will have a knowledge of clinical pathology sufficient to investigate the blood and the body fluids. How much of all these procedures he carries out himself, with his own hands or the hands of assistants, is an unimportant matter—one of time, energy and capital outlay. The important thing is for the internist to avail himself of all necessary diagnostic techniques and evaluate the findings himself, with an eye not only to establishing a diagnosis but formulating treatment. He is the conductor of the symphony who calls out the oboe and the tympanum and does not let either of them steal the show. He must see the sick person as a whole—his past and present and future, his cultural milieu, his economic background, his conflicts and worries, his emotional and intellectual assets, as well as his liabilities.

As Paracelsus, that sixteenth-century medical sage and rebel, put it: "He who wants to know man must look upon him as a whole and not as a patched-up piece of work. If he finds a part of the human body diseased, he must look for the causes which produce disease, and not merely treat the external effects." And: "The greatest and highest of all qualifications which a physician should possess is *Sapientia*—i.e., Wisdom—and without this qualification all his learning will amount to little or nothing as far as any benefit or usefulness to humanity is concerned. . . . We cannot find wisdom in books, nor in any external thing; we can only find it within ourselves."

What I have delimited as the province of internal medicine is enough for any one man. It is the nucleus, the very corpus of medicine. It differs from the field of the old-fashioned general practitioner by the recognition of its limitations and from the more highly particularized specialties by its inclusiveness.

I have not wished to cast stones at the general practitioner nor to derogate him in any way. Many of these men lead unselfish and truly heroic lives, working not a forty- or sixty-hour week but more nearly continuously, without rest or holidays or even sufficient sleep. In spite of the demands upon them some manage to keep abreast of the times; but it is a killing job. I doubt whether modern medicine can much longer be served efficiently by them.

The public is hardly yet aware that the general practitioner's day is passing and that he is being replaced not by the high-priced specialist but by the internist who should be the primary counselor in all illness. It is for him to decide when the services of a specialist are needed and to direct the crowded traffic of the sick on their road to recovery.

CHAPTER III

The Choice of Physician, Medical Fees and Etiquette

THERE is much talk today about maintaining the principle of the *free choice of physician.* No one can question the desirability of such free choice. But perhaps only among the economically more secure city dwellers does this desirable state of freely choosing one's own doctor actually obtain. The so-called middle class, or what there is left of it, the office worker and the relatively well-to-do, still depend in the main upon the services of individual doctors whom they consult in their offices or summon to their homes. In sparsely settled rural communities the choice may indeed be free but the selection is limited to the few doctors who practice there. Industrial workers often turn to plant physicians for treatment. Poorly paid wage earners and the medically indigent depend for medical care on dispensaries and hospital wards. It is perhaps better so because most of our hospitals, including the large municipal ones, require a certain minimum standard of training and experience for their staff members. The public, ignorant in such matters, is assured a certain competence and efficiency in their care which they might not receive were they dependent upon their own untutored choice. There is no point in babbling about free choice where none exists. It does not, as a rule, exist in families whose annual incomes are below two thousand dollars. In normal times more than half the families in the United States fall into this group.

On what basis is the choice made among those who can and do choose their own doctors? On what basis should it be made? The first answer is one of fact, the second one of opinion. But I have not the facts at my command, simply my impressions. They are these: It is my impression that the reasons for choosing a doctor are often quite fortuitous: Dr. Jones lives next door; Dr. Brown cured the Smith baby of whooping cough (which, incidentally, he probably did not—actually he comforted and reassured Mrs. Smith); Dr. Black charges less than Dr. Green and is just as good. I believe that most people show much more intelligence, judgment and circumspection in choosing their vacuum cleaners, their whisky and their brand of lipstick than they do in deciding which doctor to consult. My former teacher, Dr. George Sears, used to say: "A pretty good doctor is like a pretty good egg." No one wants a pretty good egg for breakfast. Now, where is the strictly fresh doctor and can I afford him at the present price of eggs? There are rules for buying horses—none for consulting doctors. A horse should be sound of wind and limb. He should stand without hitching and a lady should be able to drive him. I know some superior M.D.'s whose wind and limbs are no longer sound, if they ever were; some who are mavericks and have never been hitched; though there are many of them, to be sure, who are driven, sometimes to death, by their women patients.

In addition to what I have called the fortuitous reasons, there are others, perhaps sounder—though still in my opinion not conspicuously intelligent. "Mary has a pain in her back; there must be something wrong with her kidneys. Do you know a big kidney man?" And at the bridge table: "Dr. Blank has such a heavenly smile and such charming manners." That begins to approximate a sound basis of choice. At least it tells us something about Blank Esq., M.D. The search for the "big" man usually subsumes a previous diagnosis. Mary may have a pain in her back, to be sure, but perhaps it comes from faulty posture which is being perpetuated by her doting mama who is constantly telling her to stand up straight. Pain in the chest—big lung man. Pain in the head—big head man. Pain in the belly—big belly man. And so on ad absurdum. But it is not as simple as that. Even when there is failing vision, buzzing or ringing in the ears or a skin eruption, it does not necessarily indicate that we should go posthaste to the appropriate specialist. Perhaps these are merely symptoms of an underlying disturbance, such as diabetes or arteriosclerosis. I do not mean to imply that good specialists know only their tricks and tools. Many of them have a comprehensive grasp of the general problems of clinical medicine. I have personally known two dermatologists (skin doctors) with extraordinary diagnostic ability in the field of general medicine. That is not the point. The patient should not attempt to make his own diagnosis and then proceed according to his conclusions. He should, moreover, be in more or less continuous contact with a doctor whom he knows and trusts and who has a record of him in sickness and in health until death do them part. This doctor is the one whom the patient must choose, and having chosen him he should stick to him and take his advice until he is done with him and then he should choose another one. It is for the doctor to decide when a specialist is needed and the doctor should recommend the specialist to his patient, or several to select from if he prefers.

I am sure all this sounds like the tritest common sense, but common sense often plays an amazingly small role in the behavior of patients. When people are sick they are anxious and when propelled by anxiety, common sense flies out of the window. They hope for magic. They resort to a primitive kind of thinking. Perhaps Dr. X can do what Dr. Y cannot. "Why not try someone else?" "What was it my partner said about his doctor? He cured Mr. Lane of heart disease after everyone else had failed? Perhaps I'm going to drop dead of a heart attack as my father did when he was fifty. I've noticed that my breath is short when I climb the subway steps. Dr. Bumpus said my heart was okay, I'll go to

Lumpus and just check up on him." And so on, and so on, and so on. It simply does not make sense. Pick a man who is well trained and whom you trust. Then trust him. Don't shop around and bootleg and play fast and loose and expect miracles. All you will get is bills. If you proceed on the principle of ten cooks are better than one you will only spoil the broth of your remaining years.

Dr. David Edsall, to whom I have dedicated this book, used to say: "Eighty-five per cent of diseases anyone can diagnose and 15 per cent no one can." He qualified the 15 per cent. There are some clever or even brilliant men who can chip away at the 15 per cent and reduce it somewhat—men of great experience and learning and retentive memories, or men with noses to smell out rarities and who love them. But the great mass of medical practice deals with the commonplace: with headache, with constipation, with fatigue, with fear of disease, with fear of failure, with fear of death, with disharmony in personal relationships, with anxiety and depression and tension states or with the problems of aging and decay. The art of diagnosis is only part of the job. When your doctor is in doubt he can get help, or try to.

All this assumes that your doctor is an honest man, that he will not keep you coming back or take your money when he does not know what ails you or what to do about it. That is right. If you doubt his honesty by a jot, then drop him like a hot potato. And if you doubt the honesty of all doctors then you had better try to find out why. But if you go to another doctor to find out why, you will probably end up by questioning his honesty too.

From what has gone before you will have guessed my opinion of the proper basis for the choice of a physician. He should first of all be an internist who is well trained or who has been exposed to a good training, i.e., graduated from a Class A medical school. He should have had an internship in a good hospital and, if possible, have some active hospital affiliations, though for reasons of racial discrimination that is unfortunately not possible for all doctors. The facts are obtainable from the directory of any county medical society or from university clinics or from other doctors, preferably in noncompetitive fields. This much is sure, that stylishness and elegance, expensive equipment, attractive chintzes, stream-lined limousines, high fees and social position, membership in clubs, brilliant dinner-table conversation, even general réclame and notoriety are not in themselves hallmarks of the good doctor. He should be an honest, upright man whom you instinctively trust. He cannot always be brilliant. It is far more important that he possess integrity in a high degree. There is no one kind of personality that is the perfect one, but his personality must suit yours. I have seen excellent doctors who could pass as floorwalkers or ham actors, dapper stockbrokers, homespun farmers or ascetic saints. I know some who fraternize with their patients and others who are aloof, some with urbane bedside manners and others gruff and uncompromising. There is no patent of nobility on their sleeves. If, in addition, your doctor has wisdom and the kind of understanding that comes from suffering, and if he has tolerance and compassion, you are fortunate. The elder Oliver Wendell Holmes described a doctor who had a smile that netted him five thousand dollars a year. One of the greatest doctors I have known never smiled and almost never talked. He grunted in the laconic language of an Indian brave and patients flocked to him in adoration. There are some personalities that have a healing quality. I do not know why. As Shakespeare put it: "I have seen a medicine that's able to breathe life into a stone."

You are probably already beginning to worry about what all this is going to cost you. I have seen that look so often on patients' faces. They sit gingerly on the edge of the chair or they automatically move the chair back a little from my desk. They are thinking to themselves: "Now what have I let myself in for? What is he going to stick me?"

How often have you heard: "We can't go to Florida this winter, we've had such terrible doctor's bills," or "We'd like to turn in the car for a new one but we can't afford it; you know—that operation." Have you ever heard anyone complain of his night-club bills or his liquor bills? Have you ever heard anybody say: "I bought a magnificent pair of shoes at Stuarts' but I offered them half their price and they wouldn't come down a penny—the robbers!" What is wrong?

Night clubs, liquor, new cars, shoes represent perhaps not all durable goods but at least satisfactions. Going to your doctor probably is not one—no matter how urgent the need, no matter how Godlike a creature he may be. Besides, it is so often an unexpected expense—not on the family budget. Sometimes illness comes swiftly—like an arrow: a sudden appendicitis, a sudden pneumonia, a sudden heart attack; or it creeps in silently and stealthily, with gradual loss of weight and increasing exhaustion. Your working power is impaired, perhaps your earning capacity reduced and then the blow falls. And when you are well again you try to dismiss the whole unpleasant business from your mind —and the doctor's bill with it, as long as he will let you. No wonder many doctors have a hard time collecting their debts. But there are other explanations. To the public there seems to be no rhyme or reason for their fees. "Why, it cost five hundred dollars to have our baby; my mother paid only twenty-five for me." Jones charges fifteen dollars a visit and Harris five. Is Jones three times as good as Harris? There seems to be no yardstick, at least no recognizable one. But there is. Most doctors govern their charges by two principles. The first is time, the second is the patient's capacity to pay. Part of each day is spent for nothing—in hospital rounds or dispensaries, in teaching and attending committee meetings, in taking care of impecunious friends and relatives, in looking after other doctors and their families and in seeing patients who just cannot afford to pay. In my experience, doctors are more generous in this respect than most other professional men or businessmen. Can you imagine going into a department store and telling the manager that you are desperately in need of some new socks but you just can't afford to buy them? And would he hand you a pair? No, he would not. And yet that is just what the doctor does who sees patients in his office without recompense. Actually, each patient costs him something —a certain portion of the overhead of his running expenses. If he does not collect at least that, he will go into the red.

Doctors are, as a class, notoriously poor businessmen. They are not only generous but unrealistic and sentimental about money. They blush and stammer and say: "Oh, don't mention it—don't give it a thought." And the patients blush and stammer in a kind of competitive embarrassment. What nonsense it is. There are a certain number of working hours a day; there are a certain number of these hours in which a physician earns no money; he has a wife and children to support and life insurance to keep up and office expenses to meet. You have to pay him. And how much? That depends. If you are rich you pay his maximum fee and if you are middling you pay his middling fee and if you are penniless you pay him nothing. He may have to refer you to a dispensary unless you are too appealing or too "interesting" and then he will take you on too. Most decent doctors have a fixed maximum fee in order to deter themselves from the natural instinct of grinding the faces of the rich. Of course, there are some who are conscienceless about it, who "put in steel and take out gold," as one surgeon's activities were described. But in medicine the criteria of success are not based on what the ledger shows, as they are and should be in business.

My good friend Paracelsus, who was born the year after Columbus made his voyage, felt rather hotly about physicians who put money before their patients' welfare:

> You have entirely deserted the path indicated by nature, and built up an artificial system which is fit for nothing but to swindle the public and to prey upon the pockets of the sick. Your safety is due to

the fact that your gibberish is unintelligible to the public, who fancy that it must have a meaning, and the consequence is that no one can come near you without being cheated. Your art does not consist of curing the sick but in worming yourself into the favor of the rich, in swindling the poor, and in gaining admittance to the kitchens of the noblemen of the country. You live upon imposture, and the aid and abetment of the legal profession enables you to carry on your impostures, and to evade punishment by the law. You poison the people and ruin their health; you are sworn to use diligence in your art, but how could you do so, as you possess no art and all your boasted science is nothing but an invention to cheat and deceive? You denounce me because I do not follow your schools; but your schools can teach me nothing which could be worth knowing. You belong to the tribe of snakes, and I expect nothing but poison from you. You do not spare the sick; how could I expect that you would respect me, while I am cutting down your income by exposing your pretensions and ignorance to the public?

I have dwelt on the subject of fees because it is so closely related to what I am about to say concerning the relationship of doctor and patient, which is an intimate, personal one and should be based on a certain mutual candor. Fees often come between the doctor and his patient and unless the matter is treated simply and directly and honestly, it may interfere with his effectiveness.

And so does medical etiquette come between the doctor and his patient because patients do not understand it. They seem to look upon it as some sort of secret-society ritual. It is not. It is really very simple. It can be boiled down to this. No conscientious doctor will undertake the care of a patient already in treatment with a colleague without communicating with his colleague. Of course, if the patient says: "I'm through with my former doctor, I want to come to you now," that is another matter. No conscientious doctor will serve as a consultant on a case unless called in by the doctor in charge. That is about all there is to it. Just common-sense rules intended to protect the interests of the patient as well as the doctors.

In addition to etiquette there are certain ethical principles or standards of professional conduct to which medical men agree to conform. Some of these are provided for legally by the state licensing boards; others are matters of common consent among the members of what is called organized medicine. They have to do with such matters as refraining from advertising and soliciting, from fee splitting and from accepting rebates, and also, of course, with treating as confidential what we learn about our patients.

Most physicians have at some time taken the Hippocratic oath and to many of its articles they adhere. Of all the legacies to medicine the Oath, which appears as the frontispiece to this book, is among the noblest and most enduring. It has served generations of physicians as the banner of their ethic. Not the least remarkable of its stipulations is the one requiring of them not to gossip or divulge what they have learned, whether in practice or in their personal lives, if such is of a private and confidential nature.

Actually we know little or nothing about its author, but his name is the symbol of the perfect physician. "Each successive epoch formed a new picture of Hippocrates. Each incorporated its own yearnings in his ideal figure. What people found wanting in the doctors of their own day, they thought of as having existed in Hippocrates, who thus became a perpetual exhortation, a prick to conscience, a leader on the road to true physicianship. Along these lines he will continue to manifest his power." So the distinguished medical historian, Henry E. Sigerist of the Johns Hopkins Medical School, describes him. Perhaps my book is a quest to find him in modern clothes.

CHAPTER IV

The Relationship of Doctor and Patient

WHY is the relationship of doctor and patient of such moment? I will answer the question first and then give the reasons for my answer. Its importance lies in the fact that the physician's effectiveness, his power to heal, depends in good measure upon the inwardness of this relationship.

Perhaps I will be accused of sentimentality, of mysticism, of overweighting imponderables. Perhaps you will say: "If I have a splinter in my finger what do I care about how I feel toward Dr. X and how Dr. X feels toward me?" But if you have a splinter in your soul? If you want to die and not to live? If you need illness in order to live? If illness helps you solve the struggle of your existence? If you are the kind of individual whose emotions short-circuit and express themselves through some bodily disturbance—pain in the heart, headache, stomach-ache or irritable colon, for example—without ever recording themselves as perceived emotions, then perhaps the need for this discussion will be conceded.

But you will again fend me off. You will say: "Oh, you're talking about neurotics, about idle rich women with silver foxes and mahogany fingernails. You're not talking about me. I'm perfectly normal. I didn't come here to be psychoanalyzed." And then I will say to you: "But I *am* talking about you. You *are* perfectly normal in the sense of 'usual' [at this point you may be offended because even the most normal person does not want to be thought usual], and it's normal and usual for illness to occur in the setting of tension, of unhappiness, of frustration and of too great struggle."

Human beings are frail vessels. Life is complicated and hard. Childhood has its problems, adolescence its problems, youth and middle age have their problems, old age and decay theirs. At each point a sensitive organism reacts to stimuli from without and to impulses from within. It must maintain an equilibrium in the face of opposing pressures. If it is too rigid to adapt itself, or too responsive to withstand the onslaught of these impacts, then a "maladjustment" occurs. It usually shows itself at the point of weakest resistance.

I have just seen a young man with a pain in his middle. It is above and to the right of his navel. He is intelligent but he does not describe his symptoms with much clarity or conviction. Physical examination and X-ray investigation are suggestive of chronic appendicitis. Should he have an operation? He "would like to have it out." I learn in the course of conversation with him that he has had several depressions in his life, often coming on when faced with some difficult situation. His father and his father's father both committed suicide. I ask him, simply, whether he has ever considered suicide because I know that men so often feel that they have to follow in their fathers' footsteps. They will emulate them not only in success but in failure as well. "No," he says, "I've been through all of that. I've settled that question for myself." But has he? How do I know? And then several thoughts pass through my mind: Last week I saw another young man who had a sudden ruptured appendix and died of it. Patients given to depressions sometimes go into seriously depressed states after major operations. Depressions may conceal severe anxiety and anxiety may express itself by visceral sensations such as abdominal pain. How many mistaken diagnoses of chronic appendicitis have I seen, and how many normal appendices removed at operation? Is this patient one of those who delights to be hurt, who needs to be operated upon to satisfy some unconscious guilt, one to whom operation perhaps represents a partial suicide?

I weigh the evidence and decide that he has a diseased appendix and that it should come out in spite of the risks. Have I gone too far? Have I pried into his affairs unjustifiably? Have I simply made trouble for myself by knowing too much? I think not. His recovery and convalescence may depend in part upon my understanding of him as well as upon the surgeon's skill.

But how do we get the evidence? Do we sit him down and fire point-blank questions at him? Do we lecture to him and tell him there is nothing to be afraid of and it is silly to go into a depression anyway? Do we preen ourselves and put on our best bedside manner, with a carnation or gardenia in our buttonhole? We do none of those things.

We try to make him feel at home. We try to make him feel that we are concerned with him only. We do not answer the telephone unless it is an urgent call. And before long he is talking and we are listening. Naturally we do not let him ramble on all over the lot and waste his time and ours. We have a schedule to keep up with. To some extent we steer the conversation, usually by picking up one of his own expressions and repeating it as a question for him to enlarge upon.

In the course of such an interview something transpires. The patient reacts to being listened to with a certain half-perceived feeling, which he may indicate with look, gesture or word. What does this mean? It means, I think, this: "I am in trouble. I need help. I have found someone who cares and who wants to help me." That is the beginning of the therapeutic situation. The power and the magic are now in the doctor's hands. How are we going to use it? Everything we do from now on, every test we make, every drug we prescribe, every piece of advice we give will be fortified or perhaps vitiated by this new "thing."

What I am talking about now is a simple human experience so

common that it often goes unnoticed. It does not belong exclusively to the realm of medicine. It exists between lawyer and client, as it does between teacher and pupil, pastor and parishioner, or in any situation in which one person seeks and receives help from another. In medicine, and more particularly in psychiatry, we see the situation in "pure culture" because the seeking and receiving of help are, after all, the basis and intent of the relationship.

What is not appreciated by some doctors, though it is apperceived by their patients, is the power for good or ill that lies in this interplay of personalities. The doctor's words not only have wings but carry a charge of dynamite behind them. He had better say too little than too much and he had better choose the time and place for saying it. What is uttered in a dark room, for example, while examining a patient under the fluoroscope or looking into his eyes with the aid of an ophthalmoscope, can create a havoc of anxiety. "Well, your retinal arteries look pretty good for a man of your age; perhaps your blood pressure is a bit high. Better have a general overhauling and get your blood sugar done." Innocent words. Truthful words. But the room is dark except for one tiny piercing light, by which he is gazing into your pupil. You take it calmly enough, in a matter-of-fact way, if you're reasonably controlled. But after all you are a middle-aged businessman who smokes too much and does not get any exercise and there is a tendency to high blood pressure in your family and you are worried about the way the banks have been badgering you. Perhaps you would have been less disturbed if the words had been accompanied by a reassuring glance from the doctor in a lighted room.

For a good many years I attended "grand rounds" on Wednesday mornings. We would assemble in our white coats around some hospital bed with a chart hanging at the foot of it so that the patient could not read it. There usually was learned discourse about livers and lungs and respiratory quotients, serum proteins and urea indices. Much of it did not need to be said at the patient's bedside, but it was and is the tradition to talk about patients on rounds in their presence. Of course, the patients did not understand. What does a red-faced cop off his beat, lying in bed in a short white-cotton nightshirt tied in the back, know or care about hemoglobin? The less he knows the more he will misinterpret. What he cares about is getting back on the job or getting sickness allowance for being off. Is it *scientific* medicine to consider his liver or his bone marrow and not him? Actually one has to consider both and one is not less of a scientist but more of one for doing so, because the first task of a scientist is to observe and describe phenomena as they occur in nature. And a cop's emotions, even when off his beat, lying in bed, are none the less natural phenomena.

I do not mean to imply that physicians are thoughtless or careless. Far from it—simply that they too often do not appreciate, as their patients do, the magic and the power of their own words and acts. I have heard some excellent doctors say some amazingly stupid things. Recently a distinguished surgeon and a thoroughly kind and sensitive human being said to his patient, in my hearing: "Well, let's set the date of operation for next Tuesday or it might be too late." That was a truthful enough statement; too truthful. What he meant to say was that if he delayed much longer the operation would not do any good and the patient's malady could not be relieved by operation. But these simple words, said in the gentlest and most reassuring manner, struck terror to his patient's heart.

I recall hearing an excellent internist say to the nurse as he was leaving an ancient dowager's bedroom: "Darned if I know what's the matter with the old lady." Not only did I hear him but so, alas, did the dowager. She was incensed at being called old—though she was over eighty—and contemptuous of his crass admission of ignorance.

This leads to the moot question of whether we should tell our patients the truth and nothing but the truth. The late Dr. Richard Cabot was a zealot in this respect. I always thought him mistaken and still do. Many of my colleagues will agree with me. What appears to us to be the truth may, when pyramided by anxiety, become to our patients a distorted phantasmagoria. Stockbrokers often watch their blood pressure as they do ticker tape—it is usually better for them not to know what the daily quotation is. In the face of serious and fatal illness it is a wise rule to tell the exact facts as we see them to someone close to the patient, not only to share our responsibility but to learn his views on what the sick person should be told. People vary widely in their wish to know the worst. Some say they do and really do not. It is often a matter of nice judgment what to tell them. I have only once informed a patient that he had an inoperable cancer. He had said to me: "I want to know the facts and I've come to you because I trust you and believe that you will tell them to me." That put me on the spot, but I have usually found that the sharp wind of truth can be tempered and that patients suffering from cancer lapse into a protective state of unawareness before the death sentence is delivered.

No one can pretend to know what doctors should say or should not say. That is not the point. The point is that because of the particular kind of authority with which we are vested by our patients our words and deeds have a power enhanced far beyond the commonplace. When the president of a university confers honorary degrees on distinguished scholars his opening remarks are always the same: "By virtue of the authority vested in me." Someone or some group has granted him the power to confer honorary degrees. In much the same manner our patients grant us the power to help them recover—not, of course, by royal decree or charter or by vote of a board, but rather by their own needs. They *project* their needs onto us and we become the instruments for satisfying them. It is like any relationship in which the needs of one person are fulfilled by another who becomes thereby the embodiment of all spiritual grace and power. I am convinced, though others may not agree with me, that if there is a scattering of this energy, if it does not eventually hit its mark, if this feeling is dissipated among too many physicians, then the result may actually be a destructive one. We see it in the rich, who feel they can afford and commandeer the best medical advice and who vainly think that the next high-priced consultant or specialist will supply the panacea. We see it in the poor who are buffeted from clinic to clinic for this opinion and that opinion, and who never have the feeling that anyone is really taking care of them. And we see it in physicians themselves who usually receive execrable treatment when they are seriously sick because their colleagues are so worried about them and are loath to take on the responsibility single handed. I can think of one distinguished physician who died, I believe, because no one doctor was given the authority to help him live. This is not due to a babel of tongues or a confusion of counsel –but to a scattering of the patient's forces which should be knit together by one individual in whom the sick man has faith. When scattered they may become destructive to him. Not long ago I observed a young man in a hospital ward who was suffering from pulmonary tuberculosis. The service was not well organized. The chiefs were constantly rotating and every fortnight or so a new intern took over the care of the young man. He lost weight, became increasingly toxic and febrile, though he was given the best treatment that a modern hospital can supply. He was then sent off to the country where he was cared for by one doctor whom he immediately took to. And at once he began to improve. Was it the change and the country air? I do not think so—altogether.

I once had the opportunity of reviewing some "authenticated" case records of patients suffering from bone and intestinal tuberculosis, allegedly "cured" at the Shrine of Lourdes. What struck me as the common denominator of all of them was the fact that previous to the time the miracle occurred the suppliants had been to scores of physicians and had been given up as hopeless. When they finally emerged from the rather cold and dirty water, they received the benediction of "cure" because they could now give their undivided love to the Holy Mother. Perhaps this represents a precondition for miraculous cures.

Like Paul, in his Epistle to the Corinthians, we doctors are "made all things to all men," but still we must be above suspicion —a tall order indeed which, of course, we cannot fill. And so the relationship has always in it a kind of frustration. It is never pure. It is *ambivalent,* having mixtures of love feelings and hate feelings. It is fickle, seldom rational, though it may have the appearance of constancy and sweet reasonableness. Often we are forced to deal with a tribe of medical shoppers who are not only looking for bargains but who prefer shoddy to real goods. That is where the quack steps in and the charlatan, with their false claims and high-pressure salesmanship. For each quack there are many suckers who are driven by a need and a will to believe.

If the physician is aware of the play of these forces, if he can "take it," both love and hate, and not overreact to either, then he can utilize this relationship for his patient's good. To do that he must have some knowledge of himself, of his own feeling-life. Intuition may not be enough, though without it he is lost. Actually, I do not believe that intuition is enough. There must be, in addition, some specific training in introspection, and some experience with the problems presented by the emotions. True, a naïve but gifted physician may be far more effective than one initiated into all the esoteric writings of psychiatry, but a combination of native endowment and professional training obviously supplies the best equipment. It is like the musician; if he has absolute pitch he is at a great advantage, but an accurate ear, while essential, is not sufficient without a long period of training and self-discipline.

Much of what we, as physicians, are called upon to do is like listening to music intelligently, even though what we hear may not always charm us or soothe our savage breasts. We must be familiar with the leitmotiv. If there are thirty-three variations on a theme or a grand fugue we should recognize them as such. The art of intelligent listening constitutes a large part of the wise physician's task.

This chapter started as a kind of argument. I suspect that by now you are saying: "He can't be talking about medicine—he's talking about psychiatry." Perhaps I am talking about neither. These are, after all, academic labels. What I am really talking about is sick human beings and what they want and need to get them well. Francis Peabody, the late professor of medicine at Harvard whose too early death was a loss to American medicine, once wrote: "The secret of the care of the patient is in caring for the patient." That is certainly true. If we dislike our patients, if we allow them to "get our goats," to arouse our antagonism, it is amazing how helpless we become in helping them and amazing, too, how quickly they will sense it in spite of all of our urbanities.

But what is this practice of medicine? Is it an emotional sweat bath? Is it me and you and you and me? Is it a sentimental social service worker's dream? Is that all there is to it? Certainly not. I intimated in the beginning of this book what a rapidly expanding technical universe it has become; how the doctor has changed from Santa Claus to scientist. I am not trying to turn the clock back, but I am noting the addition of a new instrument to the doctor's medical bag—the instrument is *trained* human understanding. Without it some of our drugs and tests and gadgets may prove egregiously useless.

Medicine is not and perhaps never will be human engineering. We may know just how rapidly the blood is flowing through the kidneys and just how much urea is being cleared by them out of the blood stream per unit of time. We may know just what the stroke volume of the cardiac output is and how much reserve the heart muscle has to keep up an adequate circulation when added burdens are put upon it. We may know that in epilepsy the brain emits electrical waves of an unusual nature which can be amplified, recorded and photographed. We may know that scurvy is caused by a dietary deficiency which can be corrected by eating citrus fruits or by taking vitamin C in the form of ascorbic acid. We may know that pneumonia is caused by various races of pneumococci and that tuberculosis is caused by a bacillus of a certain size and shape which has an affinity for acid dyes and exhibits certain cultural properties.

But do we know why one man who has heart disease is an invalid and another goes about his business? Do we know why one man who develops tuberculosis dies of it and another throws it off? Do we know why one man who has been paralyzed by poliomyelitis becomes president of the United States and another spends the rest of his life sitting in the sun in a wheelchair? Is it our job not only to cure disease but to try to prevent it and to help our patients lead contented and useful lives? I believe it is. To do that we must know a great deal about them. It seems to me to be part of the problem of internal medicine to have access to that knowledge. For as one of my teachers used to say: "It is almost as important to know what kind of patient has the disease as what kind of disease the patient has."

Indeed it may be questioned whether there is any such thing as disease in the abstract. There is such a thing as a man riding home in the subway who has a sudden pain in his side and wonders what can be the matter with him. He goes home and his wife sees there is something wrong with him and turns down the bed and gets out a bottle of aspirin. He has a chill and coughs and spits up some dark sputum that looks like prune juice, and his wife takes his temperature which is 102. Then she telephones for the doctor and when the doctor comes he observes that the man's face is flushed and his pulse is rapid and his nostrils dilate a bit when he inhales and when he breathes out there is a slight audible grunt. The doctor thumps the man's chest and listens to it with a stethoscope and he discovers that just below the shoulder blade on the right side there is a patch that thumps like a boxful of sand and not like a hollow box, and that over this spot his breathing sounds not like the soft rustling of leaves but like air rushing out of the valve of a bicycle tire. And so the doctor says: "I'm afraid your husband has pneumonia."

That is pneumonia. And pneumonia is also his wife's consternation, and that unfinished brief at the office, and the doctor's bill and Jimmy's tuition. It is all of that. And the pneumococcus is always present in the mouth. What made it get Mr. Jones—just at this most inopportune moment? And that leads to another absurd question: Is there such a thing as Mr. Jones in the abstract, without the office and the tax case and the subway and his wife and their conjugal worries and Jimmy? The doctor who does his job must be in the thick of all of it. If he hopes that serum or even sulfadiazine will always do the trick alone, he may have to hope again.

Perhaps the commonest complaint that patients bring to us is *fatigue*—again not in the abstract. They say something like this: "Doctor, I don't know what's the matter with me but I seem to feel tired all the time." Well, what do we do about it? Do we go into the "surgery" and get out a bottle of nasty-tasting green medicine and say: "Here, take a teaspoonful of this three times a day before meals in a wineglassful of water. That'll pep you up"? Do we use "psychology" to suggest to him that he is not tired? Not if we're any good. We have to go to it and try to find out *why.* That is the Promethean curse under which we labor. We shake hands with him when he comes into our consulting room and if his hands are cold and clammy we have one impression. We look him in the eye and if his eyes are dull and puffy we have another impression, as we have if his eyebrows are scanty at their outer margins. If his eyes are bright and shiny and he has a pinched look about his nose we have still another impression. If his speech is slow and labored and he cannot find the words he needs, or if he is tense, fidgety and restless, we may have still another.

And then we take his history. We may begin with inquiries about his father and mother, not because we suspect that he has inherited that tired feeling but because we have gradually to reconstruct his whole existence. It may take an hour before we are ready to examine him and then at least we will know what to look for and not put him through the trouble and expense of countless routine tests. When we know him a little better we may have to ask him how he gets on with his wife or even about his sexual relations. If we ask him those things right off the bat, the chances are he will tell us his married life is one long sweet dream of love. And we may discover one of several things: that he has a deficient thyroid function resulting in a diminished oxygen consumption of his tissues; in other words, his fires are banked and the draft is shut and he cannot get up steam. Or we may find that he has an early tuberculosis, or even such an unusual disease as undulant fever, which comes from drinking infected milk. Or he may hate his job or his wife or both. Or he may be caught between the horns of some moral dilemma, or he may be running away from some inner anxiety which gives him no rest and often borders on a state of panic. Or he may be one of those souls who appear to have been born tired.

Medicine has, as yet, relatively little knowledge as to what constitutes the state of well-being. We don't know why one man is full of beans and the other one drags his hind legs; why one bounds out of bed chirruping and the other cocks a baleful eye at the miserable day. It is some subtle combination of humors or, to put it in modern terminology, it has some relation to the endocrine system: the thyroid, pituitary, the adrenals and the gonads; or to the *unconscious* mind which rides some men like an incubus and on which others seem to mount as Bellerophon did Pegasus.

CHAPTER V

Medicine and Psychoanalysis

IF THE public is confused about medicine and medical men, how much more so must they be about psychoanalysis and psychoanalysts, about psychiatry and psychiatrists. In this chapter and the next I shall try, with perhaps some temerity, to state the situation as I see it and to put these two disciplines in what I consider their proper relationships to medicine.

It is no accident that a chapter on psychoanalysis follows one on the relationship of doctor and patient. Of all of Freud's discoveries and formulations, at the pinnacle of importance is the phenomenon of *transference,* which has to do with this very topic of relationship. Curiously enough, in spite of its significance, not much of great moment has been written about it and some of its aspects still linger in the realm of unexplained mystery.

In the course of psychoanalytic treatment the patient behaves toward the doctor in a characteristic manner, characteristic for him and indeed often a kind of caricature of him. These attitudes, which may run the gamut from love and extreme dependence to resentment and hostility, are believed to be re-enactments of attitudes established in early childhood, especially in relation to parents and brothers and sisters. The patient loses, in more or less degree, the common-sense, realistic attitude of an intelligent human being seeking cure of an illness and instead shifts to a neurotic one in which childish and emotional features may predominate. From these neurotic attitudes the analyst endeavors to extricate his patient.

The art of psychoanalysis depends in large measure upon the skillful handling of the transference relationship. It exists, though in less obvious form, in all relationships between doctors and patients. As I stated in the previous chapter, much of a doctor's effectiveness as a therapist depends upon this transference situation which he uses in medical practice—unconsciously to be sure—for purposes of suggestion, persuasion and the exercise of his authority. But in psychoanalysis the physician is, or at least he aims to be, constantly aware of the transference and he analyzes its nature for the purpose of diminishing the patient's resistance to the treatment.

I have no intention of expounding psychoanalytical fact and theory to the reader. If, however, we examine the description of the transference relationship I have just given we shall discover some of the moot points about psychoanalysis.

First the words *realistic* and *neurotic;* they are now on everyone's tongue. Who would care to define them? To do so would take us into the ether of metaphysics in which we might find it difficult to breathe. It is like the color red. We recognize it even without being familiar with the wave theory of light or knowing just what the distance is in millimicrons between the crests of a light wave which looks red to us.

To be realistic is to direct one's strivings toward approximately realizable goals. To try to fly with wings of wax is certainly not so. To maneuver ourselves in such a manner as to achieve some durable satisfaction in the life of work and play and love is so. To yearn for the unattainable, to exploit suffering and illness, to be insatiable in one's hunger for affection, to be driven in spite of ourselves by unwelcome impulses, to experience undue anxiety not related to actual situations, to be torn by unreasonable conflicts, all these may be neurotic. The precise point at which they become so and a neurosis develops must rest in the end on quantitative considerations, but we have as yet no adequate tools for measuring these subtleties.

I recall a conversation with William James, the only one I had the privilege of having. It was in the days of my youth when nothing seemed beyond me. We were talking about happiness. James was a sparkling wraith who looked also like the little iron-bearded figures of men that peopled some Victorian gardens. I remember that he rubbed his stomach gleefully and said: "Happiness is *not* a bellyful of beer and sausages." So it is with these definitions. We can often only approximate the idea by exploring its negative.

Freud wrote in 1912:

> One of the invariable and indispensable preliminary conditions in *every* case of psychoneurosis is the process which Jung has aptly named *introversion* of the libido. This means that the quantity of libido which is capable of becoming conscious, and is directed towards reality, has become diminished, while the part which is unconscious and turned away from reality . . . is by so much increased. The libido (entirely or in part) has found its way back into regression and has reanimated the infantile imagos and thither we pursue it in the analytic treatment, aiming always at unearthing it, making it accessible to consciousness and at last serviceable to reality.

Having read this paragraph may I suggest that you reread it and substitute the term "psychic energy" for *libido* and "images" for *imagos.*

If "introversion of the libido" is the *sine qua non* of neurosis that does not imply that being an "introvert," to use the cliché of the day, is to be neurotic or that being an "extravert" is a sign of emotional health. This is the brand of parlor jargon that was so popular a few years ago and that happily is passing. Introversion and extraversion are probably both necessary to emotional health. I make this statement without attempting a definition of either and for the sake of dispelling the so often repeated illusion: "My husband (brother, son, not to mention my sisters and my cousins and my aunts) is a perfectly good normal American extravert—not at all neurotic." Where is this paragon of *normalcy?* And where did we get any such cock-eyed ideal of what is *normal?* Certainly not from our Puritan Fathers. Is it *normal* to put all your emotional eggs in one basket and when the basket falls to spend the rest of your life crying over spilled eggs? Is it normal to be natty and grin like a well-dressed stereotype on a billboard and think that all of life is bound up with the next bridge game or golf match or directors' meeting and never to withdraw and reflect? It has always struck me as remarkable that this boop-a-doop, jingle-jangle, boogie-woogie, they-satisfy, happiness-in-every-box civilization we have built up has retained as its imagoes two such contrasting figures as Washington and Lincoln—the one an austere, hardheaded, extraverted patrician, the other a passionate, tragi-humorous, homespun, introverted man of sorrows. And yet no careful reader of their biographies could fail to recognize attitudes of introversion in Washington and of extraversion in Lincoln.

All this leads naturally to a consideration of what is normal, another word doctors and patients often use without any clear concept in mind. In matters anatomical and physiological it is relatively easy to establish a norm on a statistical basis. To be six feet, three inches tall is not abnormal; to be a foot taller puts one in the class of a circus giant. To weigh two hundred pounds may be normal or it may not, depending on the height and the distribution of fat; to weigh three hundred pounds is abnormal. To have five million red corpuscles in every cubic millimeter of blood is normal; to have three million is abnormal. To have a blood sugar level of approximately one hundred milligrams per one hundred cubic centimeters of plasma is normal, but if it is one hundred and fifty or two hundred it may mean that one is suffering from diabetes. These are easily ascertainable standard values, derived from the examination of thousands of individuals.

When, on the other hand, we come to problems of human feelings, thoughts, emotions and behavior, we are put to it to establish any such statistically derived standards. There is so much we do not know and have as yet no way of finding out. Statistical data concerning human behavior are singularly wanting, and comparison of an individual's reactions to statistically derived standards would probably prove unrewarding, even assuming it were possible. Is it normal to eat three squares a day, to spend eight hours in bed, to marry and raise a family? Or is it normal to behave as a couple did in a modern fairy story, written by a little girl I know, which ended this way: "And so they were married and divorced and lived unhappily ever after."

No concept of normal can be separated from the cultural background of the individual. It would certainly be abnormal for Jeeves, the English butler, to kill himself because his mistress reprimanded him for burning the toast again. And yet we are told that Japanese servants are given to just such a form of self-expression. I recall a pretty young Sicilian girl who attempted suicide because her family decided they could not afford to provide her with a trousseau for her approaching marriage. Whatever the deeper causes of her impulse may have been, this was a blow to her pride and to her sense of security which she was unable to bear. No member of the Junior League or Vincent Club could behave so without exhibiting serious abnormality, but for a Sicilian girl it was not too extraordinary. To equate "normal" with "healthy" and "abnormal" with "neurotic" in any absolute sense will lead only to confusion.

We have, as yet, no satisfactory definition of a normal mind. The best we can do is to approximate one by the use of such abstractions as health and efficiency. Or we can try to exemplify it by enumerating names of great men who have exhibited intellectual vigor and creative genius. But surely such men as Leonardo da Vinci, Napoleon, Goethe and Darwin are not normal in any sense of standard or average but rather in the sense of ideal. Here is another source of confusion, for we use the concept "normal" interchangeably to represent average and ideal. In the life of the mind we are prone to think in terms of ideal values because average ones are so difficult to come by.

According to Ernest Jones "the nearest attainable criterion of normality is fearlessness," and by this he means not merely courage but the absence of anxiety and "the willing or even joyful acceptance of life, with all its visitations and chances, that distinguishes the free personality of one who is master of himself."

Here is the true Magna Carta of the mind. It is for this goal perhaps more than for any other that psychoanalysis battles. And in its struggle it has taken unto itself obloquy, misunderstanding and slander and much subversive activity. For the true moral of psychoanalysis is not license but self-knowledge, acceptance and self-mastery.

I was recently consulted by a captain in the army. He was a strapping man of forty with a rainbow service ribbon on his breast and five stars on it. He had received citations for extraordinary heroism in action in the Verdun and Meuse-Argonne offensives. There could not be much question of his courage or valor, and yet he paced the floor of my office in an agitated state, smoking one cigarette after another. His hands were cold and clammy. He was trembling. His mouth was dry.

I asked him what was the matter. He said he did not know. He was terrified. Of what? He did not know. It was all such nonsense to him. Here he was doing just what he wanted to do and yet he was panicky most of the time. When he stood up on parade ground before his company he felt sure he was going to keel over. When he went into the officer's mess he simply could not stick it: he had a feeling he had to get out. The thought of train travel was more than he could bear. And yet he was anxious for active service and not in the least afraid of combat.

He had with him an X-ray picture of his heart and an electrocardiographic tracing. He had been suffering from palpitations and a feeling of breathlessness. The heart shadow was of normal size and contour. The tracing showed a rapid rate and some extra beats. On the back of the printed tracing the doctor had written in pencil: "Tachycardia, extrasystoles, and myocardial damage." The captain wanted to know what that meant. I tried to reassure him and to explain that tachycardia was a way of saying that his heart was beating rapidly, which he knew without my telling him, that extrasystoles frequently occurred in heavy smokers, as they did in people who were agitated, and as for "myocardial damage" there was certainly no sufficient evidence for any such assumption. But his anxiety and apprehensiveness clamped onto the last, like the jaws of a vise. What did myocardial damage mean? His father had died of "myocarditis" seven years before at the age of fifty-eight. He was with him constantly until the end. He said: "I was tickled to death when he passed along, I saw him suffering so long. On the day of the funeral I was pretty much broken up. I never did really get over it but I went back to work the next day and pretended it was just one of those things. I've tried to dismiss it from my mind." The patient added that within six months to a year after his father's death he had a "nervous breakdown" and not long after that he started drinking too much.

I led him into the examining room to take his blood pressure and to listen to his heart because he wanted so desperately to be reassured that it was all right. While he was lying on the table he was seized with such terror that he begged to be allowed to get up and put his clothes back on. When he came into my consulting room he was shaking and the beads of sweat were standing out on his forehead. And yet otherwise he was the picture of health, a fine, upstanding, alert and intelligent officer.

This is the raw material of medicine. Can such a state be laughed off? Can he be kidded out of it or "there, there'd" or cured by suggestion or reassurance? I believe not. Do such conditions exist only in the idle rich who have nothing else to do but think about themselves? I am sure not. Here was a "he-man," an "extravert," a married man with three children, a success in civil life and a man with a fine military record. There was no history of shell shock in the last war, but in spite of his partial insight into his illness he felt an irrational apprehensiveness, so explosive that it seemed ready to blast him out of this one.

That the attempted cure of such a disturbance is fraught with difficulty I am sure you are ready to believe. One thing is clear: that unless we have some deeper understanding of what is going on in him, anything like a lasting cure is improbable. But how can we find out? Not by an inquisitorial attitude. Even if we knew what questions to ask him the chances are he would not know the answers. And too much questioning, pointed at his underlying problems, might actually precipitate him into a serious panic. So we proceed cautiously, with enough calm to keep him from being swamped. Such a patient will often grab onto us as a drowning man does to flotsam. He will try to press advice from us about his job, his marriage, his career, long before we are in a position to advise him. If anything goes wrong, if he leaves his wife or jumps out of a window, we shall be blamed. And if he recovers and regains his equanimity he will never want it known that he had had a "nervous breakdown," nor that he had received the benefit of psychiatric help.

And so we often hear this stock remark: "I've known many people who have been psychoanalyzed [the public sometimes prefers the vulgarism psyched] but no one who was ever helped by it. They usually come out worse than they went in." I believe that that is a misinterpretation because the facts simply are not available to the outsider.

But let us return to our handsome captain. Should he go through an analysis? Who is to say? On what basis is the decision reached? If you have a lump in your groin that transmits an impulse when you cough, it may well be a so-called inguinal hernia. Almost anyone trained in medicine can make a diagnosis. And any competent surgeon can operate on it and repair the defect in the abdominal wall. He can, moreover, tell you with a fair degree of accuracy how long you will be in the hospital, what the hospital expenses will be, how much the operation will cost you and what the chances of failure of the operation and recurrence of the hernia are. If you drive him to it he can tell you the statistical probability of accidental "death on the table" or of serious postoperative complications.

But if the lump happens to be in your throat and not in your groin, if there is fear in your heart, you may be much more disabled than you would be with a hernia. Your fear is less easily "reducible" than the hernia is. When it is pushed back it will not stay back for long. It has a way of bulging out until you are aware only of the painful mass of your fear which seems at times to strangulate your whole personality.

There is no one who can conscientiously say with any degree of assurance such as the surgeon can offer you that you will recover from your disturbance, how much it will cost you, how long it will take and what the chances of recurrence are. All that *can* be told you is this: "There is every reason to believe that you will recover from your illness. I can't tell you just how long it will be or just what it will cost you. These things usually take time—a long time. We shall have to look into the situation a little further and I'll try to decide just what you need in the way of treatment."

And so you come back to see me for a few more interviews and I study you. "Have you had anything like this before in your life and under what circumstances? Tell me something about your family—your brothers and sisters. Did you say that you felt perfectly comfortable and secure after your first visit to me? Did you say that after you left my office you felt that I was forcing you to do things against your will? You remarked that my office seemed cold and that I must be a coldhearted man." Everything is grist to the mill and yet I must not give you the impression that I am observing you in an impersonal and detached way or you will probably fly to cover. I gather information from you. When I have what I consider the necessary data I make up my mind whether your problem is suitable for analysis. There are no hard and fast rules to govern my decision, which is based on my own experience and that of others—as yet not too carefully codified. If the diagnosis is that of a neurotic disorder and there is not too much distortion of reality, not too much tendency to project your difficulties and to find an explanation for them in malign outer forces, if there is not too much impulsiveness, not too much tendency to act out your neurotic traits, if you have some insight into your illness and some genuine desire to get well, then I may decide that analysis is what you need. And when I propose it to you and tell you how long it will take you will probably demur and I may not see you again for some days or weeks. And then you will tell me you cannot possibly afford it and you will think me mercenary if I stick to a minimum fee, below which I cannot afford to take you on. And I may say to you: "If I reduce my fee beyond that you will be borrowing money from me and I prefer to have you borrow it from someone else." By that time I shall be so interested in helping you out of your mess that I shall have to guard myself against a temptation to play the benefactor and you may feel that no one else can help you but me. And I know that there are storms ahead for you, that there is no magic in this, that you will not come out of it with clean hands and a pure heart and the strength of ten. In order to create things of lasting beauty a sculptor must be willing to mess about in the clay. I know that you cannot make silk purses out of sows' ears and I certainly have no wish to make a sow's ear out of a silk purse. And you will release to me and relieve your spirit of those things that you never have mentioned to anyone else, and for days you may not be able to talk at all. And other days you will forget to show up or oversleep your hour or have important business engagements that interfere with it. If we are lucky, you may gradually become more relaxed, perhaps even more efficient. Your persistent "bad luck" may disappear and you may for the first time in your life take an interest in your children; and those damnable colds which kept you away from your work for so many days each winter may disappear or that eruption on your forehead may vanish. But where is the skeleton in the closet which you've been searching for so assiduously? You may never find hi.n. After some stormy sessions and perhaps some nightmares, which you may understand for the first time, you may reasonably expect to develop a kind of tolerance for your fear—as if you had been immunized against it by repeated small "shots." And when it is all over you may be able to say with Paracelsus: *Alterius non sit qui suus esse potest?* (Why be anyone else when you can be yourself?)

The decision about when to advise analysis is a technical one based on clinical considerations, which have to do with the structure of the personality. In making it one has to have in mind, as in any other medical problem, the probable prognosis or outcome. Are the benefits to be expected worth the time and cost? Is this the specific form of treatment indicated and are there present any important contraindications such as too great rigidity of personality, or such malignant psychopathic states as delusions of persecution? It is again like surgery. We do not operate except for specific reasons and in order to achieve specific results. Even under the most favorable circumstances, with the most complete asepsis and delicate handling of tissues, adhesions may grow. Stones in the common bile duct may form again and the sufferer may be no better off than he was. But these misadventures are not, in themselves, contraindications. On the other hand, to operate "because there is nothing else to do" is a frivolous, unsound attitude which modern surgery does not countenance. I believe that the same should be true of psychoanalysis. It is a technique devised to study, cure or alleviate certain more or less specific neurotic states. To analyze "because there is nothing else to do" has always seemed to me specious and muddleheaded.

There are often many other things to do. But the most important is *non nocere*—to do no harm. Unfortunately, in our present state of knowledge we cannot always predict and at times it may be necessary to do a kind of biopsy—a small operation, done under local anesthetic, in order to remove a piece of tissue and examine it microscopically. So we propose to our patients a trial period of a month or two, during which time we have an opportunity to scrutinize the situation more carefully.

In the Ether Dome of the Massachusetts General Hospital in Boston, where in 1846 the American dentist, William Morton, was the first to demonstrate ether anesthesia, there is, among other memorabilia, a red-plush pincushion in which the surgeons of that day kept the needles they used during operations. Today, as you know, the needles are carefully sterilized, and the nurse who hands them and other instruments to the surgeon is, as he is, rubber gloved and masked and swathed in a sterile gown. Every effort is made not to contaminate the operative field which is carefully draped.

In a sense a skillful psychoanalyst too must preserve his field of operation from contamination. He does this by a kind of studied withholding of himself from too great emotional involvement with his patients or from social relations with them. And yet if he is cold, aggressive or disciplinary he will accomplish little. The ideal attitude is one of alert, but relaxed, expectant understanding. If this is *not* the attitude and if there is too much either of tension or aloofness in the physician, his patients may be expected to react unfavorably. Psychoanalysts aim at what is called *empathy* or a feeling *into* their patients' lives rather than *sympathy* or a feeling *with* them. To be "upset" by their tragedies is no help. The skipper of a ship must not let the gale frighten him too much. He must remain calm. At times he may have to lower away, batten down the hatches and head her up to ride out the storm.

I recall a young clergyman who once consulted me because of sleeplessness. He looked careworn. He told me about some of his poor parishioners, sad tales of illness, disappointment and misery. (I have never found that the annals of the poor were either short or simple.) His heart was heavy for them. Christ had taught us that the world's sins were His sins, the world's woes His woes. My young clergyman felt it was his duty to suffer with his flock—even for them. I had the impression that he got a kind of gratification from this, a sense of virtue. I cannot believe that it is ever a *duty* to suffer or that we will lighten other people's burdens by such a degree of identification with them.

I have talked about psychoanalysis, its aims and objectives, and I have touched lightly on its technique. I should like to see this problem as well as others from the point of view of the sufferer, of the sick man. What is he to do? Where is he to go for help if he is assailed by symptoms and unhappy situations in his life which, in spite of his best will and judgment, dog his steps and repeat themselves with a humorless and inexorable insistence? Will his doctor know what to do for him? The chances are that he will use "common sense" and suggestion and treat symptoms which may for a time disappear only to recur in the same form—or another. Even the most enlightened internist cannot be expected to decide whether psychoanalysis is the method of choice, and yet only too often one hears the doctor say: "There is no situation that I cannot deal with myself. It's just a matter of common sense." If it only were. But who can decide? The psychoanalyst who is well grounded in psychiatry and not out of touch with the problems of general medicine is the logical person to make the decision. But if he has only one string to his bow and one note to his horn he will always use the same string and toot the same note and his judgment may rightly be questioned.

It is extraordinary that these problems which crosscut the practice of medicine and even surgery every day are so little understood. There are reasons for it, of course: partly the aversion that many "healthy" people have for neurotic complaints (sometimes the very ones who appear to revel in physical complaints) and partly the inadequate training in this field which medical students are exposed to even in our best schools. To be sure, there has been progress made since I was a student and an intern around 1915. In those days it was our custom to take a careful routine history and do a painstaking physical examination. If nothing was found we habitually told the patient that there was nothing the matter with him and he was sent home, perhaps with a bottle of tonic and usually with the exhortation to get plenty of fresh air and exercise. But he turned up again or went elsewhere and often became part of the crowd of restless, wandering, discontented hypochondriacs who people our clinics. Today things are different; our medical students are "exposed to psychotic material." They may be able to make a diagnosis of the major psychoses or even of such states as hysteria, or obsessional neurosis, but they are usually not taught in the medical wards or in the outpatient departments the proper handling of those conditions that may well form the bulk of their practices. They are seldom given insight into the dynamics of personality or made aware of the relationship of life situations to symptom formation. Many of them, however, evince a genuine interest in these directions, which in my own teaching I always try to emphasize.

For a complicated series of reasons—some quite irrational, if I may be allowed the paradox—most of our universities have shut their doors in the face of psychoanalysis. They have been content, as Freud said, "to warm their pot of soup at our fire," to bootleg it and dress it up in respectable form. But few of them have openly and courageously avowed its stupendous contribution to our understanding of man. This has been a detriment both to university teaching and to psychoanalysis, which has suffered from its intellectual isolation as it has from its contamination in the market place. It now needs the critique and dignity of an academic discipline. There are stirrings today which forecast such a happy development.

You may wonder why I have said so much about psychoanalysis and so little about sex. Let me say it is not for reasons of prudishness. The sexual instinct and its components constitute only part of the problem of analysis which more and more deals with the total personality in relation to other personalities and to society.

Anxiety and the defenses against it in the form of aggression or excessive passivity and submission may express itself in the social as in the sexual sphere. Wherever it manifests itself it needs to be dealt with. What do we mean by anxiety? Not fear in pure form, as in a startle reaction, but a complicated emotional structure in which the defenses against it are often more apparent than the underlying reactions. Freud has called anxiety a "danger signal" to the self. And why does it play such an important role in all illnesses? It is safe to say that almost every patient who consults us is frightened and it is often true that his fear is the most serious problem that he brings to us. He may have a headache and fear that he has high blood pressure. He may feel exhausted and fear that he has "a heart condition." A woman patient may have a pain in her breast and fear that she has cancer. Why is this so and why do our words of comfort and reassurance sometimes lay the ghost and sometimes not?

I believe the situation is something like this. There is in all of us a kind of reservoir of anxiety which is tapped when a suitable occasion arises. Depending on the head of pressure in the reservoir and the height and strength of the dam, the floodgates may either restrain it or it may inundate us. The sources of the reservoir go back to our childhood when our own helplessness, the fear of our parents, night terrors, various misconceptions and misinterpretations concerning birth and procreation, eating and elimination, fill this reservoir with a confused, rushing swirl of conflicting emotions. Perhaps even primitive and atavistic terrors contribute to it, stemming from the superstitions and fears of our prehistoric ancestors, whose truculence and blood lust, human sacrifices and puberty rites made their nights and their days hideous. The locus of this mass of anxiety or the sluice way through which it pours is the body. For if anxiety has a purpose, it exists to preserve the body from mutilation and death. And when the body is threatened by illness the waters of anxiety rise perceptibly.

All this is not to say that physical illness alone gives rise to anxiety. On the contrary the circumstances surrounding our sexual lives, our economic security, our social prestige, may be extremely productive of anxiety, but such anxiety, in the last analysis, is rooted in concern over the integrity of our bodies.

One of the most difficult experiences of man is the awareness and acceptance of his own irrationality, of the fact that much of his psychic life is hidden from him, submerged and inaccessible to reason and control. Against this unknown part he will defend himself by the use of logic. If he can explain to his own satisfaction the cause of something that he may vaguely suspect as being irrational he will feel better about it. And so if he can fix his irrational anxiety on a symptom he will not only do so, but he will often defend the symptom against all onslaughts. If the symptom is forcibly taken away from him he will fix his anxiety on a new one or his anxiety may break out in a full-blown eruption. It is for this reason that a wise physician may permit a patient the luxury of a few minor symptoms. As David Harum put it: "They say a reasonable number of fleas is good fer a dog —keeps him from broodin' over bein' a dog."

You may have guessed that anxiety does not always show its frightened face. Indeed it can be skillfully camouflaged or it may resort to all the devices of a trench warfare including going over the top with a blood-curdling yell. It is not and certainly should not be the purpose of the physician always to ferret it out and rob it of defenses which may be necessary to the conduct of a successful life. To probe and relentlessly to pursue may be the very worst thing to do, but the importance of anxiety in symptom formation must be constantly kept in mind, and treatment, to be successful, must be directed toward it as well as toward its physical manifestations or accompaniments.

For the physical manifestations of anxiety are legion and

find their expression in all the important bodily systems: the cardiovascular (heart and blood vessels), the respiratory, the gastrointestinal, the endocrine, the generative. There is no organ or group of organs that cannot be influenced by impulses from the sympathetic nervous system and these in turn are closely related to emotional states, be they sudden and acute or continuous. Whenever the caliber of a blood vessel or of a hollow organ, such as the stomach or intestines, is concerned, or the secretion of a gland, or the blood supply to the skin or the interior of the body, we are face to face with a set of conditions in which emotions may play an important part. In the chapter on psychosomatic medicine I shall discuss these problems more fully, with special reference to such illnesses as stomach ulcer, asthma and high blood pressure. It is enough for the present to point out that these are examples of illnesses in which medicine is becoming increasingly aware of the dynamic importance of the emotions. Such illnesses represent a field requiring closer co-operation between internist and psychoanalyst, or perhaps even the mastery of both techniques by one physician.

I should like now to tell a story that was recounted to me by a friend to whom the episode occurred. It will, I think, illustrate some of the things we have been discussing. He was a scientist of international reputation—a true savant, who prided himself on his great intellect, which he in truth possessed, and on his great understanding, which he did not. He was reading in bed one night when he suddenly felt a little nauseated. He got up to go to the bathroom and to his surprise vomited quite a good deal of bright-red blood. Trained as he was in the biochemical sciences he estimated roughly the volume of blood he had lost and knowing his body weight and from it the total volume of blood in circulation he realized that the loss of a cupful or two of blood would do him no harm. So back to bed he went, to resume his reading and, according to him, not in the least perturbed. But by chance he put his hand to his forehead which to his amazement he found drenched with perspiration. And then he felt his pulse which was surprisingly rapid. I believe he said it was 120 beats to the minute. This man prided himself on his stoicism and self-control. He had no awareness of the least emotional upset and had to discover it in himself as he would in another, by its objective manifestations. He was suffering from a gastric ulcer which had given him no previous symptoms.

This simple tale propounds several questions, none of which I shall attempt to answer just yet. Can anxiety or other emotions exist without awareness of them? Can they induce changes in the motility, secretion and blood supply of an organ, such as the stomach, sufficient to lead to ulcer formation and hemorrhage? I shall refer to all of this again.

This brings us naturally to the subject of awareness. We find some patients with a very much heightened awareness, others with a remarkable unawareness. Patients may become conscious of their heartbeats, as of their intestinal peristalsis, i.e., the motions of their intestines. Such reflex and more or less involuntary acts as breathing may become conscious and deliberate. Just why a shift in attention occurs is not always clear. It need not be related to structural damage and may be a reflection of concern over the function of an organ and an expression of associated anxiety. In outpatient clinics we see a great variety of reactions, not only to symptoms but to pain. We encounter men and women with large, conspicuous tumor masses which they have never themselves noticed until their attention was drawn to them. Some patients exhibit an unbelievable stoicism to procedures such as opening abscesses, while others go to pieces at the threat of a minor operative procedure. This is not necessarily an expression of their courage and fortitude. Not long since I saw an admirable and gallant young Englishman who had been through the worst of the blitz in London. He never sought refuge in a shelter but spent every night in his own bed and slept well. He had circumnavigated the globe by air and had escaped from

Singapore at the last moment. He recounted some hair-raising experiences without bravado but with that enviable and artistic understatement given to Englishmen. He looked rather seedy due to an inadequate diet. In order to do his blood count I had to prick his finger with a needle. He paled and trembled and asked if he could lie down for fear he would faint. These reactions are very primitive ones and have little to do with being chickenhearted.

I have dealt chiefly, and superficially only, with the problem of anxiety—not with such states as phobias, obsessions and character distortions, nor with rage and aggression about which so much has been written.

Anyone in practice recognizes a certain tendency to fashions in illness. It was once fashionable for women to have "the vapors" and to faint. It no longer is. We used to see the "major hysterias," with fits, hysterical paralyses, blindness, complete or partial loss of skin sensation. It was a favorite stunt of psychiatrists to demonstrate the anesthesia of an hysteric by sticking pins in him so that he looked like an unfretful porcupine. These conditions are now clinical rarities. Instead we are consulted about character difficulties, marital adjustments and problems having to do with jobs and work and, of course, about physical symptoms. Even when such complaints are part of an emotional disturbance they are in no sense "just imagination." Symptoms of this sort bring psychoanalysis and medicine closely together. For the good of our patients and for the growth of both disciplines a mutual understanding is necessary. What better place to foster such an understanding than in our universities and medical schools?

CHAPTER VI

Psychiatry and Medicine

PERHAPS it is putting the cart before the horse to have the chapter on psychoanalysis precede the one on psychiatry. Psychiatry is, of course, more inclusive and covers the whole and variegated field of abnormal human thought, feeling and behavior. Psychoanalysis is a method of investigation and treatment, which has wrought such profound changes in our comprehension of man that it is sometimes mistaken for a philosophy of life or a *Weltanschauung*. But it is not a philosophy of life. It is a technique of understanding which holds the mirror up to man's nature—and the view he has been given of himself is not altogether flattering. Like the shocking experience of catching our reflection in the three-sided mirror of the fitter's room, it shows us our too real image repeated and repeated into infinity. But actually, as we know and our friends know, we are better looking than that. Neither Darwin nor Huxley has convinced us that we are all ape—nor has even the spectacle of the contemporary world. A man's aspirations are as important as his impulses. Love and creation have never been reduced to a "nothing but" principle. To write a biography in the modern analytical mode without understanding a man's idealistic strivings is like representing him in the form of an anatomical dissection rather than of a portrait.

In many respects the study of psychiatry is the study of scientific biography. Nothing human is alien to its interests. If it has one contribution to make to medicine, and it has many, it is in its art of history taking and recording the significant events of a patient's life. Medical men often look with mixed wonder and horror at the voluminous records of psychiatrists. In the backs of their minds they are saying: "If these fellows really knew anything they wouldn't have to be so long-winded about it and they certainly wouldn't use words that we don't understand and they probably don't understand themselves." It is like the story of the man who was admiring the star-filled heavens and who remarked that he comprehended how astronomers could discover the constellations but not how they had found out their names.

Giving things names is almost the first step in scientific discovery. "In the beginning was the Word." When a child says "mama" and "papa" for the first time he is proclaiming a scientific observation, though he does not know where mama and papa come from or what their relations are to each other or to him. When a psychiatrist calls a certain disturbance of thinking and behavior "a schizophrenic reaction" he is using a somewhat poetical term to describe a series of natural phenomena which he recognizes but does not wholly understand. To understand in a scientific sense offers the eventual hope of prediction and control. Many of the problems of the organic and biological world still defy this kind of understanding. We know the cause of earthquakes and hurricanes; we can predict their advent but we are powerless to control them. Physicians, of all men, should be tolerant and patient of the acknowledged limitations of psychiatry because even in the most precise departments of their own work, scientific understanding still remains incomplete.

Empirical science begins with observation and labeling and arranging things in classes and categories, and only later does it go on to the formulation of working hypotheses and to testing these against observed fact. And still later it introduces experiment and controlled reproduction of natural phenomena. This more mature stage usually follows the introduction of new methods or of some far-flung concept which comes only to a few geniuses in a generation. The more complicated the subject matter of scientific inquiry and the greater the number of variables, the less it lends itself to quantitative study and the more difficult it will be to arrive at the stage of control and prediction. But this is no excuse for a "know nothing" attitude, or for what is as bad: forcing the material of inquiry into categories where it does not belong.

Because the cure of mental illness is uncertain and long there is a tendency on the part of the public, and of many doctors, to look for false causes and to hope that some active intervention, such as removing the tonsils or the wisdom teeth, or giving glandular injections, will bring about desired results. These procedures usually entail only a waste of valuable time. The need to "find something physical" is often insistent because it somehow tempers the bitter recognition that we are actually dealing with mental or emotional derangements.

To be sure, psychiatric investigation takes into consideration all bodily abnormalities of form and function, and no examination would be regarded as complete without careful physical studies as well. The field of psychiatry is a wide one embracing vastly dissimilar problems: the toxic psychoses due to infections or drug and alcoholic addiction; mental defects and feeblemindedness; abnormal behavior due to syphilitic changes in the brain or to arteriosclerosis; epilepsy; emotional reaction types such as melancholia or the manic-depressive psychoses; disturbances of the thinking function formerly known as dementia praecox and now, with growing understanding, called schizophrenic reactions or schizophrenia; asocial and criminal personalities and the psychoneuroses.

In all of these variegated aberrations the psychiatrist must explore the whole field of hereditary, constitutional and acquired causes and he must, above all, reconstruct his patient's life and constantly seek for repetitive patterns related to specific situations, not only in order to be able to enlarge his own understanding but also to help his patient deal with them in the future. There are times when the patient can co-operate with such an investigation and can profit from it, and there are times when he cannot. At such times facts must be obtained from relatives and friends, the sufferer himself being best treated by giving him a sense of comfort and security and reducing his acts and responsibilities to the relatively simple routine of a mental hospital. It is at such times that families grow restive and feel that nothing is being done. They ask incessantly: "When are they going to begin treatment?" and they appeal to their physicians to rescue their afflicted relative from what looks like a useless incarceration. And physicians, with the best will in the world, often make suggestions that are unwise ones because, as one of them said to me recently: "You have to say something." But the suggestions usually do little more than render the relatives impatient at a time when patience is not only a virtue but a necessity.

The question of when to advise or insist upon hospitalization is not always easy to decide. If every "crazy" person were "locked up in a lunatic asylum" the subway rush hour might be a relatively pleasurable excursion. Many of the most gifted and creative members of the community exhibit conspicuous psychopathic traits and many a simple routine job is best performed by the intellectually underprivileged.

It is my belief that physicians and surgeons should be sensitized to these problems and sufficiently educated in them to recognize the danger signals. Usually we advise hospital treatment when there is involved some risk to the patient's welfare or to that of his associates. Of course, if the probabilities of a suicidal attempt are great or if there is an outburst of violence, we have no choice. But there are other risks that sometimes require a firm decision. If the patient's home environment is such as to reinforce the process of his illness, to burden him, for example, with unbearable guilt or to foster weak and passive submission which interferes with his autonomy as a human being, we may need to recommend his removal from home. Or if an elated patient indulges in wasteful and exhausting activity, loses weight or suddenly becomes foolishly extravagant or sexually promiscuous and shows all the signs of impaired judgment, we may have no other recourse. Or again, if a depressed patient is so retarded that all he can do is sit in a chair and stare into space or so agitated that he makes his own life and his wife's a burden, we may have to recommend a mental hospital to try to break up the rut into which he has fallen. Or if the condition is one in which simple events are misinterpreted, in which ordinary sights and sounds are given special and personal significance and there are feelings of being influenced by outside forces or of being persecuted and publicly reviled, it may be so fraught with danger as to warrant an interference with the patient's usual pursuits.

Even the most resourceful psychiatrist who provides for adequate nursing care, devises routines and prescribes "occupational therapy" and sedatives, cannot always control the situation in the home environment to his patient's advantage where, it must be remembered, the seeds of his difficulty first sprouted and were nurtured. There is, moreover, a tendency to depend too much upon the use of sedative drugs which in themselves may distort and aggravate the symptoms of illness. Such simple and useful procedures as continuous tub baths or wet packs are difficult to administer at home. Home care may involve the sick man or his family in considerable expense, especially if one or more trained psychiatric attendants are needed. Indeed, the matter of expense immediately looms large in the face of these illnesses because care is often prolonged and recovery slow. Privately owned or endowed psychiatric hospitals which minister to their patients' comfort usually operate under a large overhead and consequently the cost per day must necessarily be high. The larger state institutions, excellent though they may be, naturally house a polyglot group of patients from all walks of life, whose personal comfort and individual needs must often be sacrificed just because of the weight of numbers. No wonder, then, that private patients and their families shy away from these and from our large city hospitals when the burden of mental illness afflicts them.

In addition the horror of the "lunatic asylum" still attaches to the thought of entering even a modern mental hospital, and this raises many painful doubts. "What will people say? Will he be locked up with other crazy people? Won't that have a terrible effect on him? You know he's so sensitive and so fastidious. When he comes out won't people shun him and look at him askance? Do you think he can possibly get his job back? He's so dependent on me I don't know how he'll get along unless I am there to take care of him."

Each one of these objections must be met in turn and it is best to do so in a simple, direct and truthful way. There is no disgrace whatever—any more than in entering any other hospital. The only thing to do is to look upon this as an illness and make an effort to get over it. If you broke your leg you would not try to run a race. You would be glad to have a plaster cast and a pair of crutches until the bone knitted. You need some care and protection, and freedom from responsibility for a while in order to get well. The other patients are not any crazier than you are. Part of the treatment depends on learning to get on with other people, even queer ones. Yes, the doors may be locked and they may take your personal belongings away from you until you are comfortable and less tense and less pursued by black moods and thoughts of self-injury. But as you recover you will be allowed more and more freedom. You will probably be given a regime of rest and exercise and occupation so that time will not hang on your hands and you will not brood all day as you say you have been doing. And when you come out your friends will eventually forget all about it. You may be self-conscious for a while but after you are back on the job you will soon look upon it as you would if you had had typhoid or any other illness. As for your wife and children I know how much they mean to you, but experience has taught us that people who are too worried or tense or depressed or confused, as you tell me you have been, usually seem to recover more rapidly when they are temporarily away from the ones they love most.

But if the patient flatly refuses to go to a hospital in spite of our conviction and persuasion, what is to be done? That depends pretty much on the attitude the relatives take. If they support us in our judgment we are then free to force the issue in spite of the patient's objection. Psychiatrists do not like to resort to commitment proceedings (sometimes called certification) unless it is absolutely necessary. Even the stubbornest, most recalcitrant and confused patient will often yield to persuasion if properly handled. I recall a young woman who had been lying on her bed for several days next to an open window in a locked room, threatening to jump if anyone entered. She was experiencing a kind of religious ecstasy and was quite out of contact with her environment. When the room was finally entered, through the window, she was abusive, resistant and refused to do more than pull the bedclothes up to her chin and lie stiffly staring at the ceiling. She of course resisted any effort to get her out of bed, and the proposal that she go to a hospital was met with torrential abuse. Finally she said: "At least I won't go unless you force me to"; whereupon the physician made as if to force her, taking hold of her wrists. From that moment she allowed herself to be dressed and to be carried down to the waiting ambulance.

In some states of the Union at least, it is possible to keep a patient even against his will in a licensed hospital for a period of thirty days' observation. This is a fortunate legal provision, for the first function of a mental hospital is a diagnostic one, and often prolonged observation and study are required in order to arrive at an understanding and to formulate a plan of treatment. Diagnosis is more than attaching a label for purposes of hospital statistics. It involves a deep understanding of the patient's mental, emotional and physical makeup and, above all, a conception of him in his natural habitat with all the forces of social, economic and family life impinging on him.

More even than the physician must the psychiatrist consider the patient in relation to his social milieu. And the problem of prognosis, or forecasting the probable future course of events, is of paramount importance and difficult to approach with any certainty. Both the patient and his family need to know what to expect. Will he recover? How long will it take? Will he ever be the same again? What are the chances of a recurrence of his illness? Some forms of mental and emotional disturbance are cyclical in nature: depressions and elations may recur again and again and alternate in their sequence. Naturally, the plan of a patient's whole life may be upset by these upheavals. The psychiatrist is asked to predict not only the patient's future but that of his children as well.

I am consulted by a young man whose wife has been a patient in a mental hospital because of delusions of persecution. Fear of being poisoned resulted in an aversion to food. She also exhibited personal untidiness and at times threatened the nurses. After several months she was discharged greatly improved and is now in a nursing home under the care of an excellent psychiatric nurse. The patient's younger sister has been committed to another mental hospital with a similar disturbance, perhaps even more severe and malignant. The diagnosis in both instances is a schizophrenic illness. The young husband is, of course, greatly worried. He has to be away a good deal on business. He has an excellent nurse for the children. They are living happily with his parents, who are devoted to the children. "Of course they know mummy is sick, but they don't know what's the matter with her. They keep asking for her all the time and wondering when she's coming home." The father wants above all "to do the right thing for the kids." He knows he cannot do much for his wife right now. She is suspicious of him, unreasonably jealous, and fluctuates in her attitude between extreme dependence and hostility. Her moods are quite unpredictable. The slightest thing seems to set her off.

He asks: "What are the chances of this being passed on to my children, Doctor?" And I answer something like this: "Actually, we don't know too much about heredity in relation to mental disease. We are all mixtures of good and bad traits handed down to us by our forebears. But we can do a great deal about the environment in which our children grow up. Your wife is obviously much too sick to take any responsibility for them now and the arrangements you have made for them sound pretty good to me. Do you ever write them when you are out of town or bring them presents? Couldn't you manage to spend a little more time with them and have some fun with them when you are here? They need all the sense of security they can get." Well, perhaps I have not answered his question satisfactorily but I have tried to direct his thoughts and actions into constructive channels.

But if pressed for an answer I should say something like this: The time to worry about our children's inheritance is before they are born—not after. If you have doubts about the soundness of the stock from which you come then you should subject your pedigree, as far back as you can trace it, to expert scrutiny, and your wife or fiancée should do the same. If you insist on marrying in spite of a bad hereditary load, then the one who bears it should submit to voluntary sterilization.

This does not mean that a vague history of psychoneurosis or insanity or apoplexy constitutes a bad heredity. As the British psychiatrists Henderson and Gillespie say: "The very salt of the earth may spring from such a stock." Speaking generally of the subject, they present it as "a matter that can only be approached when the public are so enlightened as to realize for themselves the difficulties, the trials and the sorrows which the propagation of defective stock means both to the parents and to the offspring." In the "free countries" all this is still left to the individual conscience, but part of the psychiatrist's job is to mold public opinion to an appreciation of its great importance. At an earlier point in their discussion the same authors remark: "There are people who do ask for help and advice in regard to marriage, but the advice given is usually acted upon only when it coincides with the applicant's own ideas."

Studies of human heredity are enormously difficult because of the time span between generations and the inaccuracy of records. Mental disturbances in which the hereditary factor is of presumptive importance are the manic-depressive psychoses, dementia praecox and epilepsy. A great deal of statistical evidence has been presented, mostly by German and Swiss psychiatrists, which indicates inherited traits in as high as 80 per cent of some of these disease groups. There are some outstanding examples of the disastrous results of the propagation of tainted stock: "Martin Kallikak married in 1837. Both he and his wife were normal, and their descendants for six generations were also normal. But Martin Kallikak had an illegitimate child by a girl who was feebleminded, and the descendants in this line in six generations in the same environment in the same State yielded 222 feebleminded out of 41 matings."

Feeblemindedness is, to be sure, often the result of brain damage due to injury or infection but there is evidence for a belief that heredity plays a determining part in some cases, as it may with genius. For example, great musical ability is said to have been present in an unbroken line through at least six generations of the male members of the Bach family. Nevertheless genius has been known to sprout and flourish in the meagerest soil, unfertilized by great forebears.

CHAPTER VII

Some Common Psychiatric Problems

THUS far I have dealt only with the more limited part of psychiatry—the psychoses, once called insanity. But there is far more to psychiatry than the care and treatment of psychotics, and it is of this aspect that I wish particularly to write. Indeed, in many respects the psychiatrist now bears the burdens of personal guidance, once the province of the old family doctor. Only in place of a benign human wisdom, or perhaps in addition to it, he has expert training and experience in dealing with the intricacies of human relationships. To be sure, often he is not consulted when he can be of most use, before habits are fixed and ruts too deeply grooved and reactions have become irreversible. Here again, as in going to a mental hospital, there clings a feeling of disgrace and stigma. Many patients fear the psychiatrist's "X-ray eyes which can see right through you," or think that "all psychiatrists must be cracked anyway." This latter conviction is sometimes shared by medical men who naturally wish to save their patients the pain of a psychiatric consultation and who will try, sometimes successfully, to deal with these problems themselves.

But by and large, practicing physicians do not have the time to deal with them, nor actually the training. Most doctors take to the woods when they run into emotionally disturbed patients. They approach them with fear or distaste or a feeling of boredom. When such attitudes prevail doctors will probably be able to do little for patients who present early signs of mental and emotional disturbance. And yet that is the very time when most can be accomplished in the prevention and relief of mental, and often of physical, illness. The whole situation is regrettable. When there is the most hope of help and prevention of disaster there is too often no one to turn to. Few of the clergy can manage human maladjustments which tax the most experienced psychiatrist. Though the confessional and absolution from sin undoubtedly furnish spiritual support and have their hygienic value, what many patients need is not forgiveness but self-understanding. By this I mean not mere intellectual insight, often enough of little use, but insight acquired in combination with an emotional re-experiencing of the pain and conflict inherent in the difficulty.

But what are all these problems that beset suffering human beings? Why do they so often need help? Our fathers and mothers got on without it and so did our grandfathers and grandmothers. What is wrong with our puling generation? Is it composed of neurotics? Is it under the spell of a guild of Svengalis who see it only in their own sickly image? And who are these psychiatrists who think they know what to do? Are they demons or demigods? Are their own lives always so serene and wholesome? "Dr. J. has been through a messy divorce himself and Dr. Q.'s child is in my daughter's class at school; I never saw such a spoiled, obnoxious brat in all my life."

The argument "what was good enough for Washington is good enough for me" has never to my mind been a cogent one. Even though Washington got along without the telephone, the internal combustion engine and incandescent lamps; without vaccination, aseptic surgery and ether anesthesia; even though he lived to a ripe old age and ended his life as he lived it, in dignity, overlooking his broad acres on the bend in the Potomac, what of the lot of the generality of mankind in his day? What of the other thousands who did not even enjoy Washington's advantages, who did not wear perukes? What of the halt, the lame and the blind, of the women who died of childbed fever, of the babies who were blinded as they emerged into the world, of the children who choked to death of diphtheria; what of the countless numbers who died needlessly of smallpox and typhoid; what of agonizing amputations and hospital gangrene; what of the insane who were put in chains and cast into dungeons? This was the medical mob scene of Washington's day. The spotlight of science has brought new figures into highlight which were previously in shadow.

Once all disease was thought to be due to the visitation of malign and evil spirits. Medicine has never wholly abandoned this view. In the realm of mental illness the thought of "possession" has survived. We know now, however, that "possession" is not from without, that people are not "hexed," but that inner forces may swamp the personality and in a sense take possession of it. Much of what in our forefathers' day was persecuted as witchcraft or the evil eye and in our parents' was reproved as willfulness or ungodliness, we now recognize as illness. The eccentric, the distracted, the maniacal, even the criminal, are looked upon no longer with the cold eye of moralistic judgment but with the inquiring eye of an observer who attempts to understand the motives and mechanisms of human behavior.

Certainly the forces of suppression have grown less. Parental authority has waned to a shadow. Traditions have worn thin. Fathers and mothers do not know what to hand on to their children except a congeries of outmoded and halfhearted convictions. Religious training and the fixed moral codes of socially homogeneous communities are far less restraining in their influences than they once were. Everything has to be thought out and experienced anew and life is approached experimentally. Man, and especially woman, has found a new freedom. The inner sources, so well damped down by the Victorians, have burst their bonds. Man has not only taken a bite out of the apple but has swallowed the whole business with a resulting colic. His new freedom and new knowledge are perhaps more than he can bear. His security is shattered. His shibboleths no longer give him free passage to a respected old age.

These.are some of the causes that account for the increase in emotional disorders. Among the causes, also, must be reckoned the fact that more people survive to maturity than did a generation or so ago, and many of these disorders appear in mid-life. With increasing responsibility and demands made upon them a disequilibrium may occur. Little wonder, then, that marriage and child rearing and work present rocks against which the waves of emotional conflict break, and that the psychiatrist is constantly called upon to deal with disturbances arising out of the tumult.

Naturally enough the psychiatrist himself is susceptible to all of the influences that impinge upon his generation. He has no God-given immunity from mental and emotional ills. Sometimes, indeed, he chooses his profession in an effort at self-cure. He is often a subjectively minded, introspective individual and he may be queer and eccentric. None of these characteristics disqualifies him if he has arrived at sufficient self-knowledge to avoid becoming emotionally caught up in his patients' problems.

I have mentioned marriage, child rearing and work in relation to all of this. Let me dwell upon them a little further. In psychiatry one cannot always separate causes and effects. An unhappy marriage can be the cause of emotional disturbance just as emotional disturbance can be the cause of an unhappy marriage. Usually both sets of conditions operate and reinforce each other. There is a tendency on the part of the public to oversimplify these matters and to say, for example, in a different context, that "So-and-so jumped from the twentieth story of the Excelsior because of the stock-market crash." If that were the sole cause, a parachute should be part of the equipment of every foresighted Wall Street man.

It is not easy to know just where to begin a discussion of the marital problems presented to a psychiatrist. He is consulted by young girls who want to get married but cannot because they are frightened, inhibited, self-conscious and overcritical; by young men-about-town who leap from one amorous encounter to another and leave a trail of cracked, if not broken, hearts behind them. They would like to settle down but they somehow do not seem to. He is consulted by married couples who hurl epithets and crockery at each other and can live neither together nor apart.

Patients come singly, in utmost privacy—sometimes even using assumed names—or, less frequently, they come in pairs. The psychiatrist must watch his step. They will try to force him into giving premature and ill-judged advice, which as often as not may be predicated on the success or failure of his own marriage. Or they will maneuver him into the position of arbiter, which is not his rightful one, or he may find himself being played off by one partner against the other. He must approach these problems with sympathetic detachment—not intent on preserving the institution for its own sake nor yet recommending divorce just because he, himself, would find his patient's situation an intolerable one. He may even be impaled on the apex of a triangle, which as like as not will be an uncomfortable seat. In all such situations he must try to find the meaning of the relationships and not deliver conventional and ex-cathedra judgments. One hears it said: "I will never forgive Dr. X for having broken up the Jones' marriage. They were such an ideal pair." Poor Dr. X! Is it really true that he broke up the marriage? And besides, how many sinking ships has he, unheralded and unsung, managed to salvage?

One of the truest things that can be said of man is that he will probably go on doing what he has been doing—unless he experiences some unusual influence, such as a religious conversion. It is only in the movies, not in real life, that people so often act contrary to their characters. Walt Disney's leopards can change their spots at will. And it is in the movies and in the fairyland of the advertising world that hubby buys a new car or Muriel opens a new brand of mayonnaise and, after years of a cat and dog existence, all is forgiven. But life is not like that.

The psychiatrist is confronted by problems having to do with promiscuity, with impotence and perversions and with all the heartache and conflict that go into some homosexual relationships. Each one of these problems is part of a larger one—the adjustment of the total personality. It is not profitable to treat the deviant sexual behavior as an end in itself but rather as a symptom of some wider disturbance. Many of these patients receive glandular injections, prostatic massage and "just plain commonsense advice" before they reluctantly find their way to a psychiatrist.

One of the commonest clichés of the day is talk about being "oversexed." That is a silly and meaningless expression. Individuals vary greatly in their sexual appetites and capacities. If there is a normal standard we do not know what it is. But certainly the ability to withstand moderate frustration is evidence of emotional stability; and an obsessional preoccupation or compulsive need is no sign of being "oversexed" but rather of a psychoneurotic disorder, often reflecting a deep insecurity in the sexual or other adjustment.

To get a so-called psychosexual history from a person requires tact and patience, and freedom on the physician's part from attitudes moralistic or prurient. No matter what his personal predilections may be, whether toward puritanism or profligacy, he must not obtrude these into the field of his inquiry if he hopes to get facts and some insight into motivation. Physicians should equip themselves, as well as their automobiles, with shock absorbers in order to travel the bumpy road of human emotions without too much discomfort.

If I were asked to state why so many marriages founder, I believe I should have to invoke modern psychoanalytical insight to find an explanation. Marriages are contracted on the basis of passion and need, and also out of certain practical considerations.

Into all human emotions and yearnings go vestigial traces of our childhood and infancy. The emotion of love revivifies these earlier patterns of thought and feeling. People deeply and romantically in love often talk baby talk to each other and find a Nirvanalike fulfillment in each other's presence which they have perhaps never known but always longed for. In so far as this normal pattern does not adapt itself to the realities of the situation and to the demands of responsibility, it is bound to lead to frustration, discontent, restlessness and even hostility. Even under the happiest circumstances some tension will exist. The balance of such forces between man and woman is tenuous and the equilibrium established is an unstable one, varying at different times of life in response to inner instinctual urges and outer circumstances. Too much denial or frustration, or infantile demands which cannot find fulfillment in marriage, may easily lead to disruption even after many years of relative contentment. This does not mean that a good marriage must be free from these elements. It is not and cannot be. Every really good wife is partly mother, sister, psychiatric nurse and courtesan. And every really good husband is partly father, brother and even mother, as well as lover. But in the midst of all of these forces there must emerge two separate individuals who walk together toward some kind of common goal, be it the rearing of their children or the comfort and respect they give each other, or their desire to take part, together, in the life of their community. If they enter into competition with each other, and even with their children, for dependent care, a tension is set up in the relationship which it sometimes cannot endure.

The modern mode of marriage puts a new strain on it. In the old home where Adam delved and Eve span, where the struggle for existence was fought out on its more primitive level, with the use of the large muscles in chopping wood and shoveling snow and dressing meat and making clothes, not only were the male and female elements sharply differentiated but survival depended on an acceptance of very real realities. In our push-button, ready-made age, survival depends more and more upon outsmarting the other fellow and keeping up a façade of respectability in the face of great insecurity resulting from circumstances beyond our control. This stirs up the waters of anxiety in us and we grasp at new straws, sometimes strangely similar to the old ones—only to founder again. But sometimes a rearrangement of forces, a more satisfied dependence or even an increased responsibility may succeed where the first attempt has failed.

Unlike other animals man is not always able to learn by trial and error. He has to find an explanation for his mistakes, as often as not by self-justification and outwardly directed blame. He cannot easily shift from one marriage to another because of habit and conscience.

The psychiatrist is called upon to guide suffering human beings through the tortured maze of their emotional entanglements, not by "telling them" with Procrustean finality, nor yet by representing to them the embodied morals of their particular cultures, which is the proper function of a minister of the Gospel. But by understanding and helping them understand the sources of their discontent he may assist them in redirecting their strivings toward more attainable satisfactions. He must winnow the kernel of health from the chaff of illness. And often, too often, he will fail in his attempt because knowledge is still insufficient and the human spirit is sticky, tough and relatively immovable.

In childhood the matrix is more plastic. Our growing knowledge has pointed with ever increasing emphasis to the importance of the first few years, even months, of life in setting the mold for future character development. "As the twig is bent so the tree inclines." Many of our psychiatric histories lead us inexorably to the nursery, to parental attitudes, to the relationship with brothers and sisters which may determine the subsequent course of a person's social behavior—and to the adolescent years when body and mind are subjected to sensations and impulses which put them to a new and sometimes devastating test.

It is a truism, none the less true, to say that what children need is food and love. When they do not get food they scream or starve. When they do not get love a number of things may happen to them. Some years ago a psychologist and his wife, similarly trained, tried the experiment of bringing up a pair of twin infants in an emotionally neutral environment. They bathed and changed and fed them with complete impersonal detachment. The scientists made careful observations and notes in utter silence, hoping to discover how a human infant developed, uninfluenced by adult provocation: when would it begin to smile, to utter sounds, to sit up, without the encouragement of a doting mother or nurse? The experiment went along famously, but before long it was the babies who turned scientists and the psychologists who were the guinea pigs. The twins put on such a show of smiling, kicking, gurgling and reaching that in the eighth month of the period of observation Mr. and Mrs. Psychologist broke down and had to call a halt out of sheer love and affection.

It may be assumed that these twins acted as they did not out of outraged sentimentality but in response to a deep inner need which found its expression and achieved its goal in an instinctive way. To be loved is no mere luxury for a child. It is as necessary for his emotional growth and development as food is for his body. And what is more—he knows it. When he is deprived of love he will instinctively try to claim it. Only his cries may fall upon deaf ears. His parents may not, because of inner conflicts of their own, be able to give him what he craves. Instead, they may, if they are in a position to afford it, engage the best nurses and pediatricians and send him to the best schools and camps and worry about the ventilation of his bedroom and about bundling him up in cold weather and seeing that his bowels move daily. All these may be expressions of love, but they also may not be. Children sense the difference. It is not always easy to love them, but if we are able to do so we can allow ourselves the luxury of an occasional temper tantrum or even a spanking without damaging them. And if we are unable to, whatever else we do for them is insufficient.

Such children often go through life with a chronic emotional hunger, always searching and never finding. They are the rejected ones who can run the whole gamut of rebellious behavior and exhibit disobedience, rudeness, temper tantrums, negativism, intellectual retardation, refusal of food, gluttony, a variety of distressing habits and tics, and even assaultiveness, cruelty, lying, stealing and delinquency. Children, not political prisoners, invented the hunger strike.

Especially in their adolescent years, children can make their parents' lives a real hell. Nothing that is done for them is sufficient. And the distracted parents ring the changes on cajolery, bullying, threats, bribery and appeasement—all to no avail—until they finally are forced, out of despair, to seek psychiatric help. To be sure, a certain degree of defiant rebellion during adolescence is a sign of emotional health. It is during this period, which may often last well into the early twenties, that parents and more often educators can help to undo some of the mistakes made earlier in the child's life. There is a tendency to avoid seeking professional advice, and yet the right word said at the right time to a troubled parent may not only relieve him of a feeling of guilt but also enable him to assume his remaining burden with more confidence.

No doubt both parents and teachers have been somewhat intimidated by psychiatrists. A simple, direct attitude toward a child is certainly one that makes for a feeling of security in him. Such an attitude now seems rather rare—at least among the educated. Many fathers and mothers no longer trust their own judgment and hesitate to act for fear of doing some harm. This attitude is in itself harmful. It is better to make mistakes than to be too uncertain and too cautious in dealing with children.

It has not been my experience, by and large, that the children of psychiatrists are happier or better adjusted than the children of more naïve parents. But in spite of this assertion, I am convinced that in the face of prevailingly hostile, nagging, or overprotective attitudes on the part of parents or of continuously un-co-operative and neurotic tendencies on the part of children, an early psychiatric consultation should be sought. It can save long periods of heartache and self-reproach and furthermore may prevent irrevocable distortion of the child's personality. Too often psychiatrists have to deal with the end results of such distortion, with a procession of unfit, asocial, withdrawn, sometimes amoral individuals.

In the age-old battle between generations the psychiatrist is often called upon to arrange the terms of armistice. To help the young or the idle or the neurotic to find a suitable occupation is one of his constant tasks. Whittling square pegs is a pretty thankless job—there are too many knots. It is sometimes easier to search for square holes. To find the right job requires not only a knowledge of aptitudes and an estimate of intelligence but some comprehension of the inner life as well. For a job well done and one to which we can bring exuberance must first of all satisfy or at least give expression to our primitive impulses. When the hounds of instinct are hot on the trail, our energies most readily overcome the irksomeness of work. Every conscientious psychiatrist has to run a kind of employment agency.

Neuroses today so often manifest themselves by work difficulties: the artist who can no longer paint, the author who can no longer write, the business executive who has lost self-confidence and decisiveness, the scientific worker whose well of ideas has run dry, the factory worker who is in constant difficulty with his foreman. And not less common is the man who cannot settle down to one thing, who has difficulty in finding himself. Sometimes this is due to a fundamental cleavage in the personality, to opposing tendencies which are difficult to reconcile.

Poets and other sensitive persons are often aware of their inner struggle. A. E. Housman has described it in himself:

The stars have not dealt me the worst they could do:
My pleasures are plenty, my troubles are two—
But oh, my two troubles they reave me of rest,
The brains in my head and the heart in my breast.

Oh grant me the ease that is granted so free,
The birthright of multitudes, give it to me,
That relish their victuals and rest on their bed
With flint in the bosom and guts in the head.

Goethe likens the split in man's soul to the bilobed leaf of the Ginko tree and again in the first part of *Faust* he says:

One impulse only are you conscious of,
O never learn to know the other state!
Alas! two souls within my breast abide,
And each from the other strives to separate.
The one, with love and healthy lust,
The world with clutching tentacles holds fast;
The other soars with power above this dust
Into the domain of our ancestral past.

The contemplation of opposites has engaged philosophers and poets for centuries. Throughout man's cultural and ethical development he has been confronted by opposing ways of thought and of life whose very opposition is resident as much in himself as in the institutions he creates. In religion we find: monotheism-pantheism, paganism-Christianity, God and the Devil; in art: classicism-romanticism; in politics: conservatism-liberalism, totalitarianism-democracy; in ethics: good and evil; in metaphysics: idealism-realism; in psychology: introversion-extraversion, aggression-submission, love and hate; in bodily structure: left and right, male and female, life and death.

These are some expressions of the duality in man's nature. They are the nutrient media on which his philosophies have fed.

Throughout civilization he has searched for a reconciling symbol, for a way of life that will synthesize and integrate his innate bipolarity. For among his strongest desires is the wish to achieve the fullness of human existence in the development of personality.

The psychiatrist is engaged in this ancient quest. Many of the symptoms with which he is daily confronted—obsessive doubt, "bisexuality," "ambivalence," for example—have their roots in this duality. There is no sidestepping the problem, insoluble as it may often be, for it seems to be part of man's heritage. As Mr. Justice Holmes said: "Continuity with the past is only a necessity, not a duty." Where there is discontinuity there can be no spiritual or emotional health. "Look unto the rock whence ye are hewn, and to the hole of the pit whence ye are digged."

If what I have said about the psychiatrist's job sounds as though he were usurping God's work—he is not. Nor have I intended to imply that he alone understands his fellow man. Such insight as Shakespeare or Tolstoy or Dostoevsky displayed is more often achieved by artists than by scientists. I have seen it in bankers and lawyers and in simple men who spend their days splicing rope, mending fishing nets and pulling lobster pots. One of Paul Robeson's songs goes:

But one thing I have got
I got an extra sense
I know what guys is like
I know what makes 'em click
I know what makes 'em tick
And when a man's O.K.
I know it a mile away.

If the psychiatrist has this insight, plus sound training and experience, he has a good equipment for dealing with some of the problems I have sketched. How he handles them will depend not only on his talents and education but also on his essential humility.

CHAPTER VIII

Psychosomatic Medicine or Mind and Body Relationships

. . . so neither ought you to attempt to cure the body without the soul; and this is the reason why the cure of many diseases is unknown to the physicians of Hellas, because they are ignorant of the whole, which ought to be studied also; for the part can never be well unless the whole is well. . . . For this is the great error of our day in the treatment of the human body, that physicians separate the soul from the body.

PLATO—more than two thousand years ago! The great ones in medicine have always known it, from Hippocrates to Paracelsus to Freud. It is just one of those truths that needs to be reiterated, retested.

Of recent years the study of the relationship of mind and body has received a fresh impetus, especially in this country. Through a growing awareness of our failures and shortcomings, through the observations of psychoanalysts, through the support given to researches by some of the foundations and through the coining of the word "psychosomatic," this whole subject has taken a new spurt. Perhaps it will appear to some as a forced growth with an insufficient root system, a showy bloom destined to rapid fading. I do not hold with this view. It is my guess that the study of the "patient as a whole" has come to stay. The reason it has been neglected during the last few decades is because doctors themselves were no longer "whole." They were so preoccupied with learning new diagnostic and therapeutic procedures that they lost sight of anything but a kind of abstract notion of disease, and they forgot in their enthusiasm that they themselves were human beings and that their patients were too.

There is a biting but humorous story by E. B. White called *The Near Demise of Mrs. Coe.* Miss Straight, the trained nurse, has just finished her lunch consisting of tomato bisque, creamed chicken, riced potatoes, romaine, huckleberry pie and demitasse. Dr. Clark arrives. Miss Straight announces to the doctor that Mrs. Coe, whose temperature has gone up to over a hundred and nine, is dead. She then hands him a sterilized ashtray for his cigarette and apologizes for having called him because Mrs. Coe's infection was localized in the throat, which is Dr. Fenway's area. Dr. Clark admits that he cannot very well encroach on Fenway's area because his own practice extends from the abdominal region to a point three inches below the knee. In the meanwhile Dr. Fenway's secretary telephones in response to a call. The doctor is at the Poultry Show at Madison Square Garden. Miss Straight again apologizes for disturbing the doctor and says: "Everything is satisfactory. Mrs. Coe is dead." Just then a nice little old man with a beard enters, wearing a long black coat smelling of iodoform and carrying a small black bag. He is old Dr. Campbell from Framingham who used to be Mrs. Coe's doctor when she was a little girl.

LITTLE OLD MAN—"Where does it hurt?"
MISS STRAIGHT—"Mrs. Coe is dead. It was a throat infection."

The Little Old Man puts on his glasses, opens Mrs. Coe's mouth with a teaspoon, peers curiously in and extracts, after a moment, a large chicken bone. Then he says: "My, my, that must have hurt."

MRS. COE (*opening her eyes*)—"Why hello, Doctor Campbell."
LITTLE OLD MAN—"Hello, Mary."

Miss Straight dips the chicken bone in alcohol and passes it to Dr. Clark, who examines it intently and remarks: "Hmm, Wyandotte. Fenway will be interested in this."

When I wrote Mr. White for permission to quote this piece he replied with this letter:

I hope you tell doctors what their job is in your book, as they seem to be working in the dark. Take a man, for instance, who has just had a major operation. His surgeon has done an excellent piece of work, really inspired cutting; the anesthetic was satisfactory and agreeable; and the patient is then returned to his bed of pain in his hospital room (the bed with the two little cranks, one for raising the head, one for raising the foot). He has also two other little cranks in the shape of a day nurse and a night nurse, perhaps, although I won't insist on that. Anyway, he is fine, all set. But on account of the modern attitude of doctors he can easily be in for the two worst weeks of his life. His old hemorrhoid has chosen this moment to pay him a friendly visit, which makes the daily enema an ordeal of the first water. Of course, he has the usual gas pains which follow an abdominal operation and his bladder and bowels have taken the week off. In addition, he seems to have a slight touch of arthritis which makes it extremely painful for him to lie in any position you can name. He is a most unhappy man and I am sorry for him. His doctor, however, is interested solely in "The Wound." The doctor shows up for a brief ecstatic moment between 10 and 11 in the morning, takes a swift look at the temperature chart to assure himself that everything is in order, whips the blanket off and peers affectionately at the beautiful scar, smiles knowingly at his handiwork, and beats it for the next victim. The inert bladder, the rheumatism, the gas pains, the nurse's curious political bias (she wants the Axis to make a separate peace with us right away so we can all unite to fight England)—all these woes which the flesh is heir to fail to engage the doctor's attention. Mention of any one of them would bore him almost beyond endurance. He is a man who has earned the right to look down from a great height on the comic spectacle of human suffering, earned it by being really good at his job, so that when he enters an abdomen he gets the organ he goes after.

I don't know, maybe it is too much to hope for, but I still hope that some day there could be a wedding between scientific proficiency and the sort of earnest solicitude and untiring sympathy of the old country doctor (when he was good). Our cold hard world of modern medicine has done strange things to the profession, and Man is taking a beating from Man.

But there is more to psychosomatic medicine than a recollection of our common humanity. It is the application to medical problems of the methods, the facts and formulations of psychiatry and psychoanalysis. It is not a new specialty or a new discipline, but an old point of view revitalized by new methods and new concepts.

Such cross-fertilization is not unprecedented in science. Actually the war on disease must be waged on many fronts. Because a new salient is opened up we need not withdraw our forces from old ones. Each man should use the weapons and the tactics that he can most successfully operate. It is only by such co-operative pincer movements that the armies of sickness and suffering and death can be cut off and surrounded.

But what does the term *psychosomatic medicine* mean? It comes from the Greek *psyche* meaning soul and *soma* meaning body. We use the word psyche to include not only the mind and the processes of thinking, but sensation and feeling and the life of the emotions as well. We are accustomed to such questionable word combinations as psychosexual and psychobiological. Psychosomatic is another of these.

Why we have named our minds or souls or spirits after Psyche is itself an interesting query. The Greek ψυχή (psyche) means breath. Throughout our language, life and breath are treated as one. We speak of dying as *expiring*. To be *inspired* means to be full of life and spirit. The Greek πνεῦμα (pneuma) as in *pneumatic*, means *wind*, also *breath* and *spirit* and *soul*. *Animal, animated* or *inanimate* derive from the Latin equivalent, *anima* meaning soul, spirit, and also air and breath. C. G. Jung has employed the term *anima* as a female representation of the inner unconscious life of man. The Greeks personified Psyche as a beautiful golden-haired maiden who fell in love with Eros or Cupid, the son of Venus. She had a great deal of trouble with her mother-in-law. The tale of Cupid and Psyche in the Metamorphoses of Apuleius is a charming and meaningful allegory. Psyche, the youngest daughter of a king, had aroused the jealousy of Venus. Venus commanded her son, Cupid, to force Psyche to fall in love with "the most despicable of men." Instead Cupid fell in love with her himself. He carried her off to a secluded spot and visited her by night. But he remained unseen and unrecognized by her. Psyche was persuaded by her sisters that her lover was, in fact, a hideous monster, in accordance with the prediction of an oracle. Finally her curiosity was too much for her. She lighted her lamp to look upon him while he slept. In her ecstasy at his beauty, she leaned over, tipping her lamp that she might look more closely at him. As she bent down, a drop of burning oil fell on Cupid's shoulder. Without saying a word he spread his wings and flew away. Psyche tried to follow him, but she had no wings and fell to the ground. Then she wandered day and night, without food or rest, in search of Cupid. Venus forced her to undertake the most difficult tasks, the last and most dangerous of which was to fetch from the underground kingdom of Pluto the box containing the ointment of beauty. She secured the box for Venus but on her way back opened it and was stupefied by the vapor. She was only restored to her senses by contact with the arrow of Cupid. Jupiter finally made her immortal and bestowed her in marriage upon her lover.

Psyche, represented in Greek art as a tender maiden with bird's or butterfly's wings, or simply as a butterfly, is the personification of the soul (both man's and woman's). She enjoys her happiness only as long as she remains unconscious. Once she lights her lamp and gives way to her curiosity, she loses her love object (as we so dryly say in psychiatry). Then follows a long period of mourning and travail and a journey to the nether world (her own unconscious). When she emerges it is again to satisfy her own "narcissism" (to open the box containing the ointment of beauty). She falls into a stupor and is aroused and restored to bliss only by the great power of love.

The symbolism of the allegory represents not only the bursting of the butterfly from the chrysalis but also the growth and maturing of man's soul through suffering and self-knowledge. It also could be used to describe the treatment of a case of anxiety hysteria by psychoanalysis in which the patient is finally able to achieve object love.

I have gone into the etymology (not to say entomology) of the word *psyche* to point out that it contains more than the notion of "mind" as a thinking machine. Almost every day doctors who deal with such matters hear some worried mother or husband or wife say: "But, Doctor, his mind is perfectly sound. You don't think he's insane, do you?" Then we have to explain that the logical faculty may indeed be sound, the memory unimpaired, and yet there may be a serious disturbance of the emotions. Many paranoid patients exhibit extraordinary shrewdness and unassailable logic, but their premises are based on fantastic and wholly unrealistic assumptions. I once knew a man who escaped from a mental hospital for a week and made three million dollars in Wall Street during his flight.

There is much evidence to make us believe that the proper operation of our higher mental functions depends upon the possession of a normal brain. Diseases of the brain such as those due to arteriosclerosis, tumor, alcoholism, lead poisoning and syphilis can produce defects in judgment and impairment of memory, of mental efficiency and of speech. They can also, of course, bring about profound alterations in the personality, changes of mood from depression and irascibility to euphoria—that happy state sometimes seen in general paresis in which the patient's outlook is unaccountably rosy, contented and optimistic.

But there are many disturbances of mood and feeling that appear to be quite unrelated to brain damage. The brain is, after all, a relatively new excrescence of the central nervous system. The instincts and emotions manifest themselves through more archaic structures: the midbrain, the spinal cord, the sympathetic nervous system, the glands of internal secretion and in our guts. Those idiots who have an undeveloped forebrain can exhibit rage, affection and, unfortunately, strong sexual impulses, just as a cat whose cerebrum has been removed by operation will fly into an undirected rage when lightly stroked and may manifest signs of sexual excitation when presented with a suitable partner.

These are examples of how disturbances of the body can influence the mind. I have already intimated, from time to time in this book, how disturbed emotions and feelings can express themselves in disordered bodily functions. There is of course, much that we still do not understand about these relationships which appear to be reciprocal. Why, for example, does a person who feels sad cry? The shedding of tears is a relatively simple physiological process. The tear glands, located in the inner corner of the eyes, are stimulated by impulses traveling down a branch of the facial nerves. This much we know. But how the mood of sadness can act as a stimulus to the nerve and thus produce a flow of tears we do not know and perhaps never will. We are dealing, as the logicians say, with two universes of discourse, the one psychological, the other physical. Each one has its own methods of investigation and its own terminology. All we can hope for, at present, are certain correlations between them. We can analyze each separately by different techniques but there remains as yet a gap in our knowledge at the point of interaction.

I remember some years ago seeing a performance of Chekhov's *Cherry Orchard* given in Russian by the Moscow Art Theater. I did not understand a word that was spoken; nevertheless the sadness and pathos were conveyed to me. I was in the company of a young actress who was overcome with uncontrollable sobbing when the governess entered the deserted and forsaken house and went through her facetious and cheering antics. One would have to know a great deal about this young actress's life to understand why she reacted so emotionally to this particular scene. But understanding the reasons for her emotion tells us nothing about the why of the physical behavior.

We are all accustomed to certain bodily responses to our emotions—indeed by definition emotions involve such responses. If we have to make an after-dinner speech, for example, our hearts may pound, our palms may be moist and our mouths dry. I have noticed that the pitcher of water on the platform is used more often at the start of the lecturer's talk than later when he has warmed to his subject. Some people are disturbed by addressing an audience—others not at all. This difference is a psychological one depending upon their personalities. To discover why would require a fairly profound psychological study which might seem to take us pretty far afield. But the character and intensity of bodily reactions are a physiological problem. Though we might be able to discover how much disturbed the speaker was by counting his pulse or measuring the moisture of his palms by a so-called psychogalvanometer (popularly known as a lie detector), we could not find out by any such means *why* he was disturbed.

In more profound states of fear the physiological disturbance may be much more intense. To put it in the words of a well-known ghost:

> I could a tale unfold whose lightest word
> Would harrow up thy soul, freeze thy young blood,
> Make thy two eyes, like stars, start from their spheres,
> Thy knotted and combined locks to part
> And each particular hair to stand on end,
> Like quills upon the fretful porpentine:

Not only the emblazoned horrors of Purgatory can elicit strong emotions of terror. I recall a young lad in a mental hospital who reacted to a distant dog bark with all the signs of intense fright. Indeed, the stimulus may often be quite inappropriate: a subway train, a cat or even a mouse. I have known stout men whose knees knocked together when first faced with a microphone, and children are often seized with fright at such innocent objects as feathers or toy balloons. Fright can be frozen in the body, so to speak. In the disease known as exophthalmic goiter or hyperthyroidism the sufferers often present the very picture of fear—wildly staring and bulging eyes, trembling hands, pounding hearts, breathlessness. The whole person seems to be "alerted" (as the army has it) for some anticipated danger. Such a state has been known to come on, in some predisposed individuals, after a sudden scare.

In rage the face reddens and becomes purple, with the veins on the forehead and neck distended. The chest heaves and the dilated nostrils quiver. We speak of "breathing out vengeance" and "fuming with anger." The body may be bent forward with the limbs more or less rigid, the mouth closed with firmness and the teeth clenched or ground together. In some instances the corners of the upper lip are drawn back and the teeth bared, which Darwin thought remarkable considering how seldom the teeth are used by men in fighting. In his classic, *The Expression of the Emotions in Man and Animals,* he says: ". . . the desire to strike becomes so intolerably strong, that inanimate objects are struck or dashed to the ground; but the gestures frequently become altogether purposeless or frantic." In the temper tantrum of the young child this undirected character of the motor discharge is what typifies it. The child will roll on the ground on his back or belly, screaming, kicking, scratching or biting everything within reach. Such behavior is symptomatically important because it represents a state of tension and frustration which finds no relief except in a somewhat self-destructive way.

Darwin points out that trembling is a frequent consequence of extreme rage. "The paralyzed lips then refuse to obey the will, and 'the voice sticks in the throat'; or it is rendered loud, harsh, and discordant." If there is much and rapid speaking, the mouth froths. The hair sometimes bristles. There is in most cases a strongly marked frown on the forehead. The eyes are always bright, with the pupils contracted, sometimes bloodshot, and are said to protrude from their sockets.

Not less accurate and observing than Darwin's pictures are some of Shakespeare's:

> But when the blast of war blows in our ears,
> Then imitate the action of the tiger:
> Stiffen the sinews, summon up the blood,
> Then lend the eye a terrible aspect;
> Now set the teeth, and stretch the nostril wide,
> Hold hard the breath, and bend up every spirit
> To his full height!

It is a temptation to go on with excerpts from Darwin. Please allow me one more—a very important one: "Most of our emotions are so closely connected with their expression, that they hardly exist if the body remains passive. . . ." And then he recounts what Louis XVI said when surrounded by a fierce mob: "Am I afraid? Feel my pulse."

Most of us, fortunately, do not often have the opportunity of witnessing the play of major emotions except on the stage or screen or in Madame Tussaud's waxworks or, perhaps, in the zoo or the nursery. Our murders are done in "cold blood," our divorces amicably arranged "between two perfectly civilized people." We cultivate the poker-face. Few of us can indulge in the luxury of gnashing our teeth or screaming without so much loss of self-respect that it has ceased to be worthwhile.

By discipline and self-control we have learned to inhibit the outer expression of our emotions, at least the action of the voluntary muscles. We cannot, however, prevent goose-pimples (the equivalent of bristling hairs) or sweating or rapidly beating hearts, for they are under the control of sympathetic nerves and involuntary muscles. Almost anyone who has sat in a dentist's chair has found that though he can prevent himself from kicking the dentist or screaming he cannot keep the sweat from gathering on his forehead.

Without the illuminating and brilliantly conceived experiments of Professor Walter B. Cannon, much of our knowledge of the bodily expression of emotions would have remained disorderly and incomplete. Cannon saw in the major emotions a kind of emergency function which prepares the body for combat or flight. Under the influence of fear, rage and pain the adrenal glands pour out their hormone into the blood stream where it is carried to various organs and through the mediation of sympathetic nerves prepares them for action. Such preparation consists, for example, of increasing the heart action, raising the blood pressure and the level of blood sugar, which is carried to the muscles and thus increases their capacity for strenuous action. There are innumerable other important by-effects.

Anyone who has seen, as I did when a medical student, one of Dr. Cannon's cats lying peacefully under a fluoroscope so that one could visualize its stomach and intestines by the use of X-rays, and then has seen the turmoil and writhing and reverse peristalsis set in motion by the mere barking of a dog, can have little doubt of the influence of fear and rage on bodily functions. The loss of control of bowels and bladder under extreme emotion is not unfamiliar.

In addition to controlling the outward expression of our emotions many of us by nature or habit or in response to anxiety have learned to suppress the associated feelings as well. It is as if, again in the dentist's chair, we not only refrained from screaming and beating up the dentist but actually experienced no pain from the business end of his drill. Immanuel Kant is said to have banished an excruciating toothache by taking thought. The extraordinary feats of certain Hindu fakirs who can walk on glowing coals probably represent some such sort of psychic deletion of pain perception. Hysterical anesthesia is a frequently encountered clinical state, though less common than it once was.

Not only can pain perception be suppressed, but so, also, can the perception of fear and rage and even love. You may recall my reference, toward the close of Chapter Five, to the stoical scientist who had to discover his own fear by observing his bodily reactions as we doctors observe them in our patients.

Why civilized man, in some cultures, has made a great virtue of concealing his emotions from himself and others would lead to interesting speculations. Perhaps it is the price he pays for civilization. When emotions find free expression hell breaks loose and man plunges into Armageddon. He has not yet found William James's Moral Equivalent of War—for the moral equivalent of war seems, alas, to be war. Man needs as much as anything a hygiene of his emotions.

Given, then, our need to control our emotions and the tendency to suppress our feelings, either consciously or unconsciously, there is often only one path left open—a discharge through the autonomic nervous system, that primitive part of the nervous system that governs heart action, respiration, the caliber of the blood vessels, the secretion of glands, the movement of the stomach and intestines and innumerable other vital bodily functions. When these become deranged by overactivity or underactivity we feel sick. And often prolonged dysfunction is followed by demonstrable structural changes. Doctors then say that the patient has an organic disease. But there is no clearly established point at which a functional disturbance becomes organic. It is, indeed, no longer a useful distinction and it is one that medicine is gradually abandoning.

Let me now summarize briefly my views on psychosomatic medicine. I do not look upon it in any sense as a new specialty or indeed as a specialty at all. It is essentially sound clinical medicine which takes the *whole* patient into account. The facts and theories derived from psychoanalysis have been largely responsible for awakening interest in this field and for illuminating it. Sometimes I have thought that, like Kipling's mule, psychosomatic medicine was "without ancestry or hope of progeny." But actually it has a venerable ancestry, stemming from Aristotle. The quality of its progeny will depend, as in all other departments of science, upon careful, considered and painstaking work—and also upon some hard conceptual thinking. There is a dualism in the name which does violence to nature. The mind and the body are one. To see them stereoscopically requires a greater understanding than we as yet possess.

CHAPTER IX

Stomach Ulcer

SOME people can "eat nails." Others are habitually dyspeptic; they look at a tempting meal with misgiving and they keep their bicarbonate within easy reach. They love cabbage but cabbage does not love them. Their stomachs are their weak spots. When they are tired or worried or unhappy it is their stomachs that kick up first.

Without any expert knowledge, just from everyday experience, we can say quite a lot about such people. We might guess that they would be spare rather than fat, inclined to be sensitive and pessimistic, reserved rather than expansive, perhaps a little irritable and tense.

Language bears out this description. The word *hypochondria* stems from the Greek *hypo* (under) and *chondros* (cartilage), especially that of the breastbone or ribs. This anatomical region which includes the stomach was formerly supposed to be the seat of melancholy and "vapors." In the singular form (hypochondrium) the word was once used as an expression for general depression, melancholy or low spirits. But in modern psychiatric usage, as in the word *hypochondriasis,* it has lost its anatomical implication and now refers to that unhappy state of mind in which there is over concern with the body and an unfounded conviction and fear of disease.

The notion that there is a relationship between mood and midriff (once thought to be the seat of the soul) has clung to medicine. Clinicians still point out that patients with pulmonary disease, such as tuberculosis, are inclined to be sanguine and cheerful and that those with affections below the diaphragm are more usually gloomy.

A more intimate and penetrating psychological study of the lives of many patients with stomach ulcers has brought to light important facts about them. Apparently they suffer from certain characteristic conflicts which they are usually unable to resolve. The man who appears outwardly to be a hard-driving, active, efficient go-getter proves actually to be a hungry, dependent person whose unsatisfied cravings for love he is unable to accept because he feels them to be too humiliating. They do not correspond to the picture he has of himself. He tries hard to compensate for his essential weakness. Indeed he has a tendency to overcompensate it. When his ambition is thwarted or his efforts toward success and accomplishment and leadership are too strained he will have a tendency to run for cover, to slip back into a dependent, childlike attitude, to put his thumb in his mouth, so to speak. Now there is reason to believe that these passive, receptive, thumb-sucking cravings when not satisfied—as they can hardly be in such an upstanding he-man—and when continually repressed, actually find their expression in a primitive way. Just as anger and fear and pain may express themselves in the form of trembling and pallor and sweating, so the need to be loved and cared for, especially when denied, may express itself as a desire to be fed. The stomach is then constantly "alerted" and behaves as it does in hunger.

Dr. Franz Alexander, who has studied patients suffering from ulcer by the psychoanalytical method, formulated an hypothesis which experimental work done by others has in the main supported. Here is an admirable example of the insight to be gained even into mechanical and physiological processes through careful psychological study. Alexander's views are based on the knowledge that the craving for love and care, when unsatisfied, can be felt *as if* it were a need for food, to which the body then reacts with a kind of chronic hunger. Such a state keeps the stomach in continuous preparedness for food which it does not receive. Its muscular wall contracts, resulting in gnawing sensations and hunger pains; its mucous membrane becomes engorged with blood and its acid-secreting glands work overtime.

There are, to be sure, other ways of reacting to such severe emotional privations. Some persons gorge themselves and grow fat, as if to make up for what they have missed. Others in defiance and spite go on hunger strikes. But there appears to be a type of individual in whom the stomach itself is the chief organ of emotional expression and in whom ulcer is liable to occur.

One of Alexander's patients, a married man of forty-six, was described as "not at all the leader-type," but on the contrary his attitude lacked the usual ambition so frequently found in persons suffering from ulcer. He remained always mediocre in his profession. He was married to an extremely able, intellectually superior, active woman, who in no sense mothered him. She devoted her life entirely to the promotion of her own career and he, being thwarted in his need for care, was driven into a competitive attitude toward her. Unlike many ulcer patients he did not enjoy his responsibility, but detested the ambition and effort to which he was forced by his wife's superiority. During eighteen years of marriage he suffered from chronic hyperacidity and pain which came on a few hours after eating and was relieved by food. Then came the ulcer. Two years later, when at the peak of his conflict, he suffered from a severe hemorrhage. This patient subsequently cured himself. He entered into a relationship with another woman of a motherly type, the exact opposite of his wife. His wife never would cook for him, he complained, but this woman did. She was a nice, soft woman who did not drive him into unattainable ambitions. He could live with her the modest life he had always longed for; and with her his stomach was at rest and he was free from symptoms.

It may seem a far cry from marital unhappiness to laboratory studies performed on dogs. I have in mind certain experiments in which an artificial opening was created at the end of the esophagus so that the animals were given sham feedings. The food which they bolted never entered the stomach at all, but fell to the floor instead, where the dogs snapped it up again and went on eating greedily for some time. The result was a powerful stimulation of gastric secretion and motility in the empty stomach which led regularly to ulcer formation.

The great Russian physiologist Pavlov proved that the secretion of saliva and of gastric juice could be sharply conditioned not only to the smell of food or to a definite feeding time but also to such signals as the sounding of a bell or of a metronome. Indeed, the salivary gland can be trained to secrete when the metronome beats at the rate of sixty per minute, but not at a slower or a faster one.

Our knowledge of the gastric juice stems from an extraordinary episode in American medical history. It concerns William Beaumont, a surgeon in the United States army. Beaumont was born in Lebanon, Connecticut, in 1785 and died sixty-eight years later at St. Louis where he had a busy surgical practice. A veteran of the War of 1812, the truly important day in his life was June 6, 1822. He was then stationed at Fort Mackinac, in Northern Michigan Territory, where a small detachment of United States troops was installed to keep the Indians in check and to do police duty on the frontier. On this particular June day hunters and trappers in the employ of the American Fur Company were returning to the trading post with laden canoes. An eighteen-year-old voyageur named Alexis St. Martin was standing in the company store when suddenly a shotgun was accidentally discharged. The muzzle was not more than two feet from St. Martin's body. Dr. Beaumont was immediately sent for and thought that St. Martin could not survive thirty-six hours. Actually he recovered from his seemingly mortal wound, married, had four children and lived to the age of eighty-three. In a "Memorial" presented to the Senate and House of Representatives Beaumont stated:

> The wound was received just under the left breast, and supposed, at the time, to have been mortal. A large portion of the side was blown off, the ribs fractured and openings made into the cavities of the chest and abdomen, through which protruded portions of the lungs and stomach, much lacerated and burnt, exhibiting altogether an appalling and hopeless case. The diaphragm was lacerated and a perforation made directly into the cavity of the stomach, through which food was escaping at the time your memorialist [*sic*] was called to his relief. His life was at first wholly despaired of, but he very unexpectedly survived the immediate effects of the wound, and necessarily continued a long time under the constant professional care and treatment of your memorialist, and, by the blessing of God, finally recovered his health and strength.
>
> At the end of about ten months the wound was partially healed [but St. Martin was] altogether helpless and suffering under the debilitating effects of his wounds—naked and destitute of everything. In this situation your memorialist received, kept, nursed, medically and surgically treated and sustained him, at much inconvenience and expense, for nearly two years, dressing his wound daily, and for a considerable part of the time twice a day, nursed him, fed him, clothed him, lodged him and furnished him with such necessaries and comforts as his condition and suffering required.
>
> At the end of these two years he had become able to walk and help himself a little, though unable to provide for his own necessities. In this situation your memorialist retained St. Martin in his family for the special purpose of making physiological experiments.

The article of agreement in which St. Martin bound himself to Beaumont for a term of one year in return for board and lodging and the sum of $150 is itself of historical interest both in form and content. St. Martin contracted to:

> Serve, abide and continue with the said William Beaumont, wherever he shall go or travel or reside in any part of the world his cove-

nant servant and diligently and faithfully, etc. . . . that he, the said Alexis, will at all times during said term when thereto directed or required by said William, submit, to assist and promote by all means in his power such philosophical or medical experiments as the said William shall direct or cause to be made on or in the said stomach of him, the said Alexis, either through and by means of the aperture or opening thereto in the side of him, the said Alexis, or otherwise, and will obey, suffer and comply with all reasonable and proper orders of or experiments of the said William in relation thereto and in relation to the exhibiting and showing of his said stomach and the powers and properties thereto and of the appurtenances and the powers, properties and situation and state of the contents thereof.

Not for one year but intermittently for eight, Beaumont became the Boswell of St. Martin's stomach, recording studiously its comings and goings, its fillings and emptyings, by observing these through the permanent hole in his side which opened directly into the stomach. The work was published in Plattsburg in 1833 under the title *Experiments and Observations on the Gastric Juice and the Physiology of Digestion.* A facsimile edition was reprinted in 1929 on the occasion of the XIIIth International Physiological Congress held in Boston, at which time a medal was struck in honor of this intrepid and single-minded scientist. As a foreword to the facsimile edition an address by Sir William Osler, delivered before the St. Louis Medical Society in 1902, is included. Osler lists the most important of the results of Beaumont's observations. Among them he enumerates the physical and chemical description of the gastric juice; the recognition that the important acid was muriatic or hydrochloric, that mucus was a separate secretion; the comprehensive and thorough study of the motions of the stomach on which most of our present knowledge is based; a study of the digestibility of different articles of diet as, for example, soured tripe, pig's feet, wild goose and venison steak, and the establishment by direct observation of the profound influence of mental disturbances on the secretion of the gastric juice and on digestion.

It is with this latter "psychosomatic" aspect of the stomach's behavior that we are particularly concerned in the present chapter. To get the information we need we must leap over one hundred years. The time is the present, the scene a laboratory in a huge, complicated, highly endowed modern metropolitan university clinic, the characters a professor of neurology and his man Friday, known as Tom. Instead of the romantic, high-collared, Empire-style tunic of an army officer of the middle 1800's that Beaumont wore, Dr. Harold Wolff wears a long white coat. Tom is dressed in a laboratory assistant's olive-drab coat, not in a mackinaw and fur hat such as Alexis St. Martin no doubt had on when he received his historic wound. But if you remove Tom's outer covering you will find that he, too, has a hole in his stomach through which Dr. Wolff can peer and take samples of gastric juice and make temperature measurements just as his illustrious predecessor had done. Tom was not shot in the stomach. The hole was made by a surgeon. It had to be. When he was nine he drank some scalding-hot clam chowder which so burnt his esophagus that it closed up. Dr. Wolff says of him:

> Since then he has fed himself through a gastric fistula 3.5 centimeters in diameter, surgically produced shortly after the accident. It is his custom to put food into his mouth and, after tasting and chewing it, to expectorate it into an ordinary kitchen funnel inserted into his stoma [opening]. . . . The patient is in excellent health, has rare digestive complaints. He is a small wiry man of forty-seven, of Irish-American stock, unschooled, married and the father of one child. He is shy, sensitive, proud, stubborn and slightly suspicious. He is fun-loving but very conscientious.

Sometimes Tom has a pint of beer. He takes a mouthful, spits it out and pours the rest of the bottle directly into his stomach through the funnel.

Given this subject's rather tense, sensitive and reactive nature and Dr. Wolff's interest in body-mind relationships, the combination was ideal. He found that emotional disturbance was accompanied by profound alterations in gastric physiology. When, for example, Tom's hostility or resentment or anxiety was aroused the lining of his stomach would quickly become engorged and red, just as would his face. He got hot under the belt as well as under the collar. There was a sharp acceleration of acid production and vigorous muscular contraction of the stomach wall. But when suddenly frightened Tom's face would become pale and there would be an accompanying pallor of his gastric mucosa and a fall in the rate of acid production and a decrease in motility.

I am sure there are French proverbs that tell us not to eat when we are tired or sad or angry. However, we do not need to be guided by proverbs, because we usually lose our appetites under such circumstances or suffer from indigestion if we do eat. It is more than estheticism that has introduced candlelight and soft music into the dining room. Good companionship and cheerful conversation are excellent appetizers and digestives.

But Dr. Wolff's experiments have gone far beyond the obvious. He has observed that prolonged increase of acid secretion in the stomach, however provoked, whether by emotional or other stimuli, results in a suffusion of the mucous membrane that lines the stomach. A kind of deep blushing takes place. When the stomach lining is in this engorged state it is unusually susceptible to injury; even the most trifling damage results in hemorrhages and small erosions. Ordinarily the lining is protected from injury by an effective coating of mucus. When an engorged, eroded area of the stomach's lining is deprived of this protection and is constantly bathed in acid gastric juice the result is the formation of a peptic ulcer. Dr. Wolff has actually produced such ulcers in Tom's stomach but he did not allow them to continue for more than four days, when by applying a protective dressing he was able to observe complete healing within three days. Indeed, physiologists have often wondered why the stomach wall is not digested by its own gastric juice. It is not digested because under normal circumstances the gastric juice does not gain access to it, the lining of the stomach being normally covered by an efficient insulation.

Here, then, is an admirable example of the painstaking, meticulous work of an experimenter putting to the test hypotheses derived not only from common observation but based on psychological inquiries into the intricacies of man's emotions and personal relationships.

Undoubtedly our knowledge is still far from complete and the mechanism here described may be only one of many, but the cause of ulcer formation and its proper treatment are certainly more clearly understood than they were. Gastroenterologists are now far more attentive to the emotional setting of their patients' lives than they were and they are daily impressed by the fact that control of diet and administration of alkalies are not alone sufficient to cure ulcers.

Indeed, a strange situation is arising. Being impressed with the importance of emotional features, these specialists now occasionally refer a patient suffering from ulcer to a psychiatrist. This usually comes as a kind of shock to the patient, who arrives at the consultation bewildered and frightened. I saw one such person recently. He was fidgety and ill at ease. At the close of the interview he said: "Gee! I didn't know it was going to be like this. I thought you would hypnotize me or give me one of those new drugs and get me to tell you something terrible about myself!" Actually we had discussed his habits of life, his family situation and his work. He was one of those eager, efficient men always in a hurry, always ahead of time, never satisfied with himself—a hard player and a poor loser. He loved to putter around the house. When he painted a wall he was never quite pleased with the results. There were too many brush marks, or the color was not to his exact liking. I think one can say of such a person, not that he complains of his stomach but that his stomach complains of him. I am sure that the two can sometimes be helped to live together on better terms.

What I have said about the stomach certainly holds true of the intestines as well. That our emotions frequently express themselves in the behavior of our guts is common knowledge, and it is now generally agreed that in such ailments as colitis and constipation the emotional factor must be dealt with. Though the physiological and perhaps the psychological mechanisms may be different from the ones we have just considered in relation to the stomach, we are interested here in certain general principles rather than in a specific mechanism.

The modern world with its hazards and uncertainties, with its blitzes and blackouts, has put a great strain on man's emotional life. The need to be heroic is more than many can bear. That there has been an increase in stomach trouble, and that ulcers have been responsible for many draft rejections and for much invalidism in the fighting forces and the civilian population, is not surprising in view of what we now know.

CHAPTER X

Allergy, Asthma and Tuberculosis

ONE morning I was preparing to give a patient some anti-pneumococcus serum. He was a man of about forty, not very sick. He had a small involvement of one of the lobes of his lungs. It was early in the disease, about the second or third day. A specimen of his sputum had been "moused," that is, injected into a mouse, and the washings from the mouse's peritoneal cavity had shown the presence of Type I pneumococcus. He was, therefore, a suitable case for serum treatment, especially since the illness was at its beginning. Before inserting a needle into his vein to inject the serum, I tested him for his sensitiveness to horse serum, since the serum he was about to get was obtained from the blood of horses, themselves immunized by injections of pneumococcus cultures. To make the test for sensitiveness I diluted some sterile horse serum ten times by the addition of a sterile salt solution. Of this highly diluted solution I injected $1/10$ cubic centimeter or one small drop into the skin of my patient's arm, intending to see whether in the next half hour or so a wheal or hivelike reaction would develop at the site of inoculation. But I did not have to wait long to discover that he was sensitive to horse serum—and violently so. He turned a slaty blue gray, the color of wet ashes, he gasped for breath, his pulse was imperceptible and he was drenched with cold perspiration. He was suffering from allergic shock and was revived by the rapid injection of adrenalin, which I had ready at hand. Had he been given the serum directly into the vein without this preliminary test he would probably have died. Actually he made a good recovery without benefit of serum.

This curious phenomenon was discovered accidentally and independently by two great scientists—the French physiologist Richet and the American bacteriologist Theobald Smith, although before them Magendie, in 1839, and Simon Flexner, in 1894, had stumbled on the same thing without realizing its importance. It is so with scientific discoveries. The time must be ripe for them to find their proper place.

Richet was studying the toxicity of eel serum in dogs. The story goes that there was a shortage of dogs in Richet's laboratory and he was forced therefore to use them for several successive injections. He then discovered that the second injection, when given a certain length of time after the first, often proved fatal, whereas the first had been relatively innocuous. Richet spoke of this phenomenon as "anaphylaxis" to express its antithesis to prophylaxis or protective inoculation.

Theobald Smith was injecting guinea pigs with diphtheria antitoxin (which, like pneumonia serum, is derived from horses). He noticed that the guinea pigs which had been injected acquired great susceptibility to normal horse serum when another injection was made several days later. These guinea pigs had become sensitized to the serum. When a sensitized guinea pig receives a subsequent injection after a suitable period of incubation a characteristic train of symptoms follows. After a few minutes the guinea pig appears to be restless and uneasy, and will usually rub its nose with its forepaws. It may sneeze and cough. At the same time it breathes rapidly and the fur will appear ruffled. After a while the animal is seized with great weakness; it falls to its side and there is irregular twitching of the legs. The respirations become slow and shallow and the thorax remains in a more or less expanded condition in spite of strong inspiratory efforts. Frequently in this phase general convulsions set in and in these the guinea pig usually dies. The lungs of such an animal after death are found to be distended, completely filling the thorax. The condition of the lungs is due to a contraction of the small bronchioles which practically block the air passages, so that little or no air enters the lungs in spite of violent respiratory efforts. The contracted muscles of the bronchial tubes imprison the air in the lungs, which therefore remain after death in an expanded, noncollapsible state like a blown-up toy balloon. The entire picture is reminiscent of that seen in a patient suffering from a severe attack of asthma.

We sometimes see patients scratch their noses after receiving an injection of some foreign protein just as guinea pigs do. Fortunately, due to our testing for sensitivity and to the taking of careful histories, we are able to avoid fatal accidents. But once one has seen a severe allergic shock in a human being one is not likely to forget it.

Why was my patient allergic to horse serum? We do not know the answer. He may have had an injection of antidiphtheria serum or antitetanus serum (also obtained from horses) earlier in life, but not necessarily so. But we do know that he had somehow been sensitized by some exposure, just as individuals may be sensitized to ragweed or goldenrod pollen or eggs or fish or cheese or house dust or wool or cats or dogs or chocolate or a hundred and one other things. If they are sensitive to these substances, then subsequent exposure to them may produce a variety of symptoms: fits of sneezing or coughing, or stuffiness of the nasal passages or attacks of asthma, or skin reactions such as itching, urticarial eruptions (hives) or eczema.

When I was in France during the last war we had at our hospital a stable of Percherons that were used for work on the grounds. It was customary to order a detail of men to police the stables and currycomb the horses. The company commander selected among others for this duty a lad who claimed that he suffered from horse asthma. Since army officers all come from Missouri ("I suppose you're allergic to dishwashing and potato peels too!"), I was ordered to accompany the soldier to the stable to supervise his currycombing. No sooner did the horse dander begin to fly than he was seized with an agonizing asthmatic attack which produced almost as much consternation in me as it did in him. He was *allergic* to horse dander.

The word *allergic* is of recent origin. It was introduced into scientific literature in 1906 by the distinguished Viennese pediatrician von Pirquet. It derives from a combination of two Greek words *allos* (other) and *ergon* (work), the whole meaning *altered force*. One hears so much of allergy these days that the public has taken up the word in a general way to describe almost any sensitiveness ("My husband is allergic to work"; "My boy seems to be allergic to soap and water"), but actually it has a very specific meaning and refers to certain altered reactions to substances to which the tissues have been previously exposed. It was formerly believed that these substances all belonged to the class of proteins, but recent observations have proved that exposure to much simpler chemicals, such as aspirin, may lead to allergic reactions.

A patient of mine recently had a troublesome case of hives from the prolonged use of the new drug sulfadiazine. He said to me: "Doctor, I'm ashamed of this skin of mine. I guess it's one of those allergic things—the kind that nervous women get who can't wear fur pieces or silks without breaking out." But why nervous women? We shall come to that presently.

Let me digress and turn back a few centuries.

In 1552 John Hamilton of Edinburgh, Archbishop of St. Andrews, was in a very distressful state of mind and body. He was forty years old and for ten years he had been suffering from asthma. He had advised with his personal physician and had consulted the royal physicians at the courts of Francis I and of Charles V of Spain. But he was getting worse. The disease, he was told, was due to a cold moist brain; a distillation of phlegm accumulating in that organ discharged itself through the wind pipe into the lungs, causing cough, expectoration and dyspnoea—as well it might. The Archbishop decided to call to his help Jerome Cardan, then Professor of Medicine at Pavia, and the most celebrated physician of Europe.

Cardan was celebrated not only as a physician. He was a mathematician, astrologer and poet as well. A charming and vivid account of his journey to Scotland and his sojourn there was given by the late Dr. Charles L. Dana in "The Story of a Great Consultation."

Apparently Cardan thought that the archbishop's brain instead of being cold and humid was hot and dry, causing humors distilled in the stomach to rise to the brain. The archbishop was, in fact, a great eater and drinker and took no exercise; he worked hard, kept irregular hours and was not shy with the ladies. Cardan prescribed a strict regime of rest, fresh air, exercise and diet just as we might do today, with some minor modifications. He neither bled him nor purged him nor prescribed a great variety of useless drugs in the manner of his time.

The archbishop was to rise at eight and take a shower bath once a week, the first ever taken in Scotland. He was then to take a quiet walk in a shady place, chewing a little mastic, the sixteenth-century substitute for gum. This caused expectoration and helped to purge the brain. At nine o'clock he was to have breakfast consisting of liver with a little ginger and some bread with two ounces of white wine. After this he could have a little chicken and a little more wine. Then he was to rest and amuse himself. From twelve to four he was allowed to attend to business but was forbidden to write letters with his own hand. At four an hour's ride on horseback was ordered. Then he could hold an audience. Supper at seven o'clock was like breakfast but preceded by a teaspoonful of honey, and additional articles of diet allowed were turtle soup, snails, barley water and chicken broth. He was to retire at half-past eight and get ten hours' sleep. There were other specific directions for purging the head which included stroking it vigorously with an ivory comb. He was to drink a quart of milk a day and as a laxative to use preserved peaches and sugar of violets.

Cardan forbade the archbishop to sleep on a feather bed and made him use a linen pillow. Today when asthmatics are sensitive to goose feathers we give them pillows stuffed with horsehair or with some material that does not pulverize, or we advise the use of a specially prepared pillowcase that prevents feather dust from coming through. Of course, we do not know that Archbishop Hamilton was in fact allergic to goose feathers. Surely that would have sounded as fantastic to his physicians as some of their theories do to us. But we know that the reverend gentleman recovered after Cardan's treatment, which is suggestive evidence of an allergic state with perhaps an accompanying chronic sinusitis to boot (phlegm from the brain). Curiously enough, Dr. Dana does not comment on the feather bed and pillow. It was brought to my attention long ago by the late Professor L. J. Henderson.

There is another element in this interesting story which perhaps deserves consideration. Dr. William Cassinate, the archbishop's personal physician, had failed to help him even after consultation with the two most famous doctors of Paris. When Cardan was invited to come, "he thought England immensely cold; that the grass was full of worms and the sky darkened with crows." When he finally arrived in Edinburgh (it took him twenty-three days to get there from London) he kept his patient waiting forty days before beginning his treatments. In the meanwhile he allowed Dr. Cassinate to carry on with the advice acquired from the Parisian consultants, who had never seen the sick man. Archbishop Hamilton grew more and more restive and finally demanded that Cardan take over. In this way did the famous Cardan prepare his ground.

Cardan was, moreover, a man touched with genius, with perhaps a dash of madness and charlatanry: a great gambler—had he not written a treatise on the evils of gaming?; a devotee of music which he lamented as a sign of weakness; a believer in omens and a lover of cats. One day his cat despoiled the manuscript of his "Lecture on Medicine," then dragged it from the shelves to the floor, leaving untouched his "Book on Fate." Cardan accepted the cat's judgment and resigned from the university.

In advising his patron he counseled him on sexual matters in spite of the injunctions of the church. This part Dr. Dana modestly leaves in Latin. Is it possible that so experienced and colorful a man as Cardan had a pretty good appreciation of his patient's psyche and was able to relieve him of much anxiety? That he understood the English character seems probable from this comment: They "care little or not at all for death. . . . Cheerfully, without blanching, without tottering, they bear with constancy the final doom."

Can it be that the mind or the emotions can play a part in such an illness as asthma for which, as we have seen, there are often chemical incitants? What would you say to this? A man who could not bear the climate in Silesia, where he suffered from severe asthma, moved away to a place where he was free from symptoms. While away he received a letter from Silesia urging him to return. This was enough to precipitate an attack. Another patient regularly had a severe attack of asthma at five o'clock in the afternoon. One day in the course of an animated conversation he missed his regular attack. When his attention was called to it he took out his watch, grew quite pale and began to gasp. It was seven o'clock. There is a report of a case of a person whose asthmatic attacks were always associated with stormy weather. An attack was precipitated when his wife suggested to him that a landscape he was looking at in an art gallery "had almost the mood of your stormy weather." I am indebted to Dr. Thomas French for these examples which are taken from his monograph on "Psychogenic Factors in Bronchial Asthma," to which I shall refer again presently. But perhaps the most impressive example is that of a patient who was sensitive to roses and who developed an attack when he was presented with a paper rose.

These instances must impress anyone with the great complexity of the problem of allergy. Today all thorough students of the subject realize the importance of emotional factors in determining the "threshold" of sensitivity. Psychotherapy can often reduce the frequency and intensity of attacks or banish them altogether, even without removal of those substances that had previously produced attacks. For example, a woman, after psychoanalytical treatment, was able to eat chicken, corn and cabbage freely and could tolerate the presence of dogs and cats, all of which she had been unable to do before.

There are many cases reported of asthmatic attacks coinciding with periods in which the patient was subject to severe emotional conflicts or was disturbed by anxiety resulting from a variety of frightening experiences. Dr. French has tried to drive an entering wedge into this knotty problem by subjecting a number of asthmatic patients to psychoanalytical study. He has emphasized the great importance of confession in the psychotherapy of the chronic asthmatic.

Other forms of allergic responses such as hay fever and various skin eruptions have been less carefully studied from the psychosomatic point of view than has asthma, yet there can be little doubt of the importance of psychological factors in connection with them. The skin is related to the central nervous system not only embryologically but perhaps psychologically as well. By color and texture it reflects our moods and our state of well-being. Compare the pink, elastic cheek of youth with the sallow, sagging parchment of extreme old age, or the ruddy glow of health with the pasty, doughy look of sickness. By our blushing and pallor and sweating we betray our emotions.

How often have I heard a patient say: "Why, doctor, I've never had a blemish on my skin in my life before!" There is a pride in our integument, as though a perfect skin revealed a perfect soul. I have seen hardheaded businessmen greatly concerned over some scarcely noticeable eruption on the forehead. The pimples of adolescence are too often connected in the mind with "secret vices" of youth, and boils are thought to be a concentration of deep-seated corruption coming to the surface.

A moralistic attitude toward purity and health has survived in folk medicine, which has never quite shaken off its animistic cloak. Such an attitude is in part responsible for the enthusiastic use of spring tonics to "clean out the blood," for dosings with calomel, for the miserable laxative habit, and for the popular ritual of the high enema—and no doubt has boosted the manufacture and sale of cosmetics to a major industry. Beauty may be only skin deep, but not so purity.

No wonder that such concepts as "autointoxication" and "too much acid" take hold of the popular imagination. What notion could be more congenial to the contrite heart than the thought that we are always poisoning ourselves. "If thine eye offend thee, pluck it out"; and so out with the teeth, tonsils, uterus, ovaries, appendix or anything that is removable. It is wonderful how medical thought has been influenced by just such Old Testament doxies.

Take "acid" for example. Most patients talk about acid as though it were something evil and corroding. They must be full of acid because they have some red blotches somewhere. They can't eat grapefruit or oranges because these fruits are "too acid," which actually they are not. They contain citric acid, to be sure, but in such form that they leave, after digestion, a residue of alkali in the body. The blood and body fluids are provided with buffer substances which permit the ingestion of large quantities of acid foods without in the least altering their reaction, which is wonderfully constant. It is only at the point of death, or in certain severe diseases such as diabetes, or after prolonged starvation, or in pernicious vomiting that a condition of acidosis arises, or in certain disturbances of metabolism such as gout, when crystals of uric acid are deposited in the joints. But to the average layman acid is bad and alkali is good. I have never heard a patient say he is "rotten with alkali" or that he must have alkalosis—which, incidentally, is just as harmful as acidosis. I once helped save the life of a woman who had poisoned herself by taking (on medical advice) a teaspoonful of bicarbonate of soda each day for a month. She retained it all and enough water to come pretty near drowning in her own body fluids. She had a severe alkalosis. We kept her alive in an oxygen chamber and stopped the bicarbonate. She lost forty pounds in two days.

But I was talking about the skin. Closely related to asthma are certain kinds of eczema and other skin affections which, like asthma, appear to be related to emotional states. In neither of them can the psychological element be properly looked upon as the *cause* of the illness. But it is often contributory, tipping the scales toward illness in an otherwise predisposed individual. For this reason some form of psychotherapy may be of the greatest help.

Turning now to the even more obscure problem of the emotions in relation to tuberculosis, I should like to begin with two case histories:

The first concerns a young European girl of aristocratic origin and background who made up her mind against her parents' will to go to a university. She had always been a somewhat shy, reticent, easily depressed child, readily inclined to tears and rather solitary. There were many difficulties at home. The parents were not happily married. There was much friction in the atmosphere and little love, although her mother was constantly concerned with her daughter's welfare. The girl had outspoken artistic interests. She loved music and the theater, and had a respectable talent for drawing. She was, on the other hand, greatly interested in languages—wavering between the two interests. This was a source of conflict not only in her but between herself and her parents. Finally after much indecision she decided to pursue the study of languages and only after long persuasion and against great resistance could she win her parents' consent. They were by no means liberal with her in financial matters so that she lived at the university in modest isolation. In the course of the second semester she began to realize that academic work was not giving her the release and satisfaction she had hoped for. Naturally this made her very unhappy but she tried with all her might to push through her plan of study, if only not to be upbraided by her father. She dragged along until the close of the semester hardly able to follow the lectures properly.

During the holidays she returned home only to hear reproaches because she looked so bad and because of her moods. She was sent to a doctor who could find nothing wrong with her. She was constantly assailed by doubts as to the wisdom of further pursuing her studies. After a most unpleasant scene with her parents she became depressed and then began to cough. Another physical examination was negative, but her cough persisted. Upon returning to the university she consulted a specialist who at first could find no evidence of disease in her lungs, but repeated examinations and X-ray studies disclosed an incipient tuberculous process at the tip of her right lung.

The second case concerns a man in his early thirties who enjoyed not only excellent health but a happy marriage and good financial circumstances as well. His wife was a young and charming woman—also apparently in perfect health. During her untroubled pregnancy he pursued his usual business activities and hobbies. He was an active sportsman and even rode in steeplechases. His wife's delivery was a difficult one and shortly thereafter she began to fail from what subsequently proved to be a malignant growth in her uterus. Her illness lasted about a year when she died. He had not given up hope of her recovery until a few weeks before the end, and in spite of his intense worry he continued in good health. As soon as the hopelessness of her condition became clear to him, however, he began to feel bad, became depressed and lost his joy of living. After his wife's death his depression grew worse. Within a few weeks he spat up some bright red blood, which he did not relate to a disease of the lungs because such a possibility did not occur to him. Upon examination the diagnosis of early tuberculosis was established.

These two stories, though striking, are by no means unusual. They are culled from many such. An extensive medical literature has recently sprung up in this field under the subheading: "Mental Aspects of Tuberculosis." One observer has found that in a hundred patients there were thirty-four in whom emotional disturbance "apparently undermined" their resistance to the disease and whose illness was "apparently of an advanced type on this account."

What does this mean? "I thought tuberculosis was *caused* by the tubercle bacillus." So it is. Its discovery in 1882 by the great German bacteriologist Robert Koch was one of the milestones of modern medicine. But the tubercle bacillus, though ubiquitous, has not yet inherited the earth. Man's resistance to it is such that he has managed to survive. Many of us have undoubtedly had slight infections which we were able to combat by our natural processes of immunity. The evidence for this statement rests on the fact that both X-ray studies and autopsy findings in many adults show healed tuberculous scars in the lungs, and on the additional fact that almost all adults give a positive reaction to tuberculin when it is injected into the skin.

Many elements play a determining role in the onset of infection. Among them must be counted not only the mass and virulence of the invading organism but the resistance of the "host" as well. Exhaustion, fatigue, cold and hunger, chronic disease, alcoholism, all play a part in lowering resistance. Scientific evidence has not yet been furnished to prove that emotional states can depress bodily resistance to infection or influence the cellular and chemical reactions involved in immunity. But the presumptive and empirical evidence is fairly convincing. One need not wait upon proof before formulating working hypotheses. If one did, scientific progress would soon become frozen. Galilei is reported to have said that ignorance had been his best teacher; for in order to overcome it in his opponents he had been driven to a variety of experiments, which he would not have performed to convince himself alone. A great contribution to psychosomatic medicine could be made if it could be proved by carefully controlled observation that immunological processes are altered by emotional states. Such proof is not yet at hand. This chapter of medicine has not yet been written.

Besides tuberculosis the resistance to other infections, such as pneumonia, influenza, sinusitis, tonsillitis and even to common cold, is probably influenced by emotional states. Again there is no proof. But everyday observation of children and adults brings the probability home to us. We need, above all, carefully recorded data so that these casual observations may be investigated by the methods of science.

CHAPTER XI

High Blood Pressure

IF YOU should accidentally gash your wrist deeply the blood gushing out of the cut radial artery would spurt about five feet into the air. The height of this column of blood would be a measure of your blood pressure. But fortunately we do not need to sever an artery in order to make such measurements. We do it by the simple device of placing a pneumatic rubber cuff around the arm and inflating it to a point where it compresses the main artery sufficiently to obliterate the pulse beat. It is similar to putting a tourniquet on the arm. Having obliterated the pulse we gradually deflate the cuff to a point where the beat is just able to come through and we then read the pressure in the cuff, either on a scale next to a column of mercury or on the dial of an aneroid barometerlike instrument. In either case the blood pressure is expressed in millimeters of mercury, just as barometric pressure may be. Simple as this now sounds to us, it is worth recalling that blood-pressure recordings in man were not made until the beginning of this century. The new methods and knowledge were the result of Italian, English and German researches done in the decade 1896–1906.

In 1733, long before this work was done, an English curate and physiologist named Stephen Hales

caused a Mare to be tied down alive on her Back, she was fourteen Hands high, and about fourteen Years of Age, had a *Fistula* on her Withers, was neither very lean, nor yet lusty: Having laid open the left crural Artery about three Inches from her Belly, I inserted into it a brass Pipe . . . and to that . . . I fixed a glass Tube . . . which was nine Feet in Length: Then untying the Ligature on the Artery, the Blood rose in the Tube eight Feet three Inches perpendicular above the Level of the left Ventricle of the Heart. . . .

It is difficult for us to appreciate what a sealed book the study of blood pressure in man must have been before the now familiar devices were introduced into common clinical use.

Of recent years instead of feeling for the return of the pulse with the fingers the stethoscope has been used to detect it. This method has proved more accurate. It gives us, moreover, not only the so-called systolic blood pressure but the diastolic as well. The contraction of the heart is called systole, whereas its relaxation or dilatation is called diastole. During the heart's contraction the pressure of blood in the arteries is naturally higher than during its dilatation because an added column of blood has just been squeezed into the pipe lines. But even when the heart dilates and sucks blood from the great veins into itself the arterial system remains full and the blood in it is under pressure, due partly to the elasticity of the arteries themselves. This prevailing head of pressure in the arteries is known as the diastolic pressure. Though usually unfamiliar to the layman, its measurement is as important as the systolic pressure, perhaps more so. The two values together give us a rough estimate of the efficiency of the circulation and of the load that the heart and blood vessels are carrying. It is customary to express them in the form of a fraction such as $^{120}/_{70}$, in which the upper figure represents systolic pressure and the lower diastolic.

"Doctor, what should my blood pressure be? They tell me it's 100 plus my age." This formula is as simple as it is inaccurate. The truth is more like this: From childhood to puberty the level of blood pressure gradually rises, attaining the approximate adult level in the period from seventeen to twenty years. There it stays till about forty when it has a slight tendency to rise with increasing age and weight, but on the average not more than 15 millimeters.

Of the two figures the diastolic is the more constant, the systolic the more fluctuating, varying with conditions of rest and activity, sleep and wakefulness, illness and health and, of course, as is commonly known, with excitement, anger, fear and other emotional disturbances.

For many years doctors have recognized that people suffering from high blood pressure or hypertension are inclined to be nervous and tense. Indeed, the most successful method of treating them has consisted of a regimen of rest and relaxation combined with the use of sedatives. We tell them "to stop worrying," "to forget it and take it easy" or "to go for a short holiday." But in my experience it is seldom true that a man will "forget it" just because his doctor tells him to; and many men when ordered to go away for a holiday take their worries with them. The direct question "Is anything worrying you? Have you anything on your mind?" seldom elicits a useful answer. Worry is an elusive troglodyte that lives and breeds in the hidden caverns of the mind and cannot easily be ferreted out. He must be coaxed and cajoled. He will show his real face only when he feels reasonably secure. Usually we can at first catch only a glimpse of his mask. What appears on the surface to be "business worries" may actually have to do with domestic relations, and these in turn are often the extension and continuation of attitudes acquired in childhood toward parents and brothers and sisters.

So the direct approach "Is anything worrying you?" is usually met with a negative reply. There is one thing we can be pretty sure of: if the patient *knows* that his blood pressure is "up," he is probably worried about that. He is aware of the fact that so-and-so was refused life insurance because of high blood pressure or was rejected for the draft, or his own father dropped dead of "a heart condition" when he was only forty-five, or he has an aunt who had a stroke and "whose blood pressure was so high it nearly blew the top of her head off."

It is fairly generally recognized that high blood pressure is associated with disease of the heart and arteries and kidneys and that it often leads to chronic illness and invalidism. Thus knowledge of its existence often produces consternation and anxiety in a person already, by nature, tense and anxious. We must dole out information guardedly and not permit our patients to watch the fluctuations of their blood pressure as they would stock-market quotations on the financial page. For in many respects this is a different problem from those dealt with in the preceding two chapters. Such illnesses as peptic ulcer or bronchial asthma speak to the patient. They draw his attention to the particular organ system involved. If he has heartburn or nausea or vomiting he blames his stomach, or if he awakens in the middle of the night wheezing and gasping for breath and all choked up he blames his old "bronichal tubes," as clinic patients prefer to call them. But hypertension is a general disease involving an organ system of which the sufferer has no awareness. For no one is conscious of his arterioles, which constitute the finer twigs of the arterial tree; and when they become chronically constricted, as they do in some types of hypertension, no special sensations are necessarily experienced.

Many physicians accidentally discover high blood pressure in patients who come to them for routine checkup or who suffer from minor complaints that usually are not related to their circulatory system. Patients do not complain of high blood pressure. They may complain of the fact that they fear its serious consequence; or, more likely, they will speak of headache, nervousness, irritability and fatigue. Sometimes they may complain of numbness and tingling in the fingers and toes or of a sense of pressure and constriction in the chest or of blurred vision, but these symptoms seldom appear until the diseased state has been in existence for some time and usually not until it has been discovered in the course of a general examination.

We have as yet no certain knowledge of the pathological process that promotes the narrowing of the finer arterioles and hence the rise in blood pressure. In many instances, at least, some interference with the blood flow through the kidneys is probably in part responsible. Opinion and evidence as to the importance of the kidneys in relation to hypertension have gone through many changes and fluctuations during the past few decades. Just now they are again in the forefront, owing to the convincing and beautifully executed animal experiments of Goldblatt, who has produced in dogs a disease quite analogous to that occurring in man by artificially creating in them a partial constriction of the artery supplying one kidney. The kidney thus partially deprived of its normal blood supply is thought to elaborate chemicals known as *pressor substances* which raise the level of the general blood pressure. If interference with the blood supply to a kidney is permitted to persist the dogs will exhibit changes characteristic of human malignant hypertension: gradual enlargement of the heart with evidences of heart failure, loss of efficiency of the kidneys as excretory organs and even inflammatory and hemorrhagic changes in the eyes. But if the clamp on the artery supplying the kidney is removed in time, the dogs' blood pressure will be restored to normal. So it will be if the artery is entirely, instead of partially, occluded or if the kidney, the blood supply of which has been experimentally reduced, is surgically removed. All these facts point to the production of pressor substances by the impaired kidney. There is an increasing body of evidence in favor of the view that some such substances occur in the natural disease of man. But the problem is far from simple and is further complicated by the fact that prolonged hypertension and constriction of the arterioles bring about pathological changes in the kidneys which may then be the result as well as the cause of the elevated blood pressure.

There are, to be sure, elements other than the kidneys that may be responsible for the origin of this puzzling and challenging illness. Influences remote from the kidneys may affect the blood flow through them as, for example, nervous stimulation and the secretion of adrenalin. These, in turn, may be the result of emotional upsets. Indeed, the physiologist Homer Smith and his associates have supplied a valuable link in the chain of evidence by demonstrating that blood flow through the human kidney is greatly reduced during acute anxiety states. Here again there is good reason for inquiring into the emotional problem associated with hypertension, even were it not for the histories which our patients give us.

Such biographical facts are not too easily come by. A very special kind of interview is required in which the question and answer method is not rigorously adhered to. When possible, a good relationship with the patient is fostered and the narration of his life history is allowed to flow in any way he wishes, without emphasis on chronological order. After the material is thus gathered it is rearranged chronologically and an effort is made to understand and interpret the main tendencies of the patient's life. When one studies sufferers from high blood pressure by such a method certain patterns of behavior, common to most of them, become apparent, although the events of their lives and their cultural backgrounds may be vastly dissimilar.

What emerges are certain kinds of emotional conflict situations which these patients seem never able to resolve. By and large they are unable to accept either their strong passive dependent attitudes or freely to express their hostile impulses. They live in a state of civil war resulting from these two attitudes blocking each other and producing a kind of emotional stalemate. This situation is, to be sure, true of many neurotic individuals as well, but the latter often succeed in resolving their problems, to some extent at least, by the development of hysterical or other symptoms. Not so the hypertensive. Although many of them develop evanescent symptoms that might be called neurotic, and frequently exhibit states of anxiety and depression, on the whole the battle seems to be fought out in the body and culminates with the development of high blood pressure. There is certainly a very definite relationship between the struggle that goes on in these patients' lives and the development of their illness—though I do not wish to be understood by this remark to make the claim that their emotional struggle is the sole cause of illness. It most assuredly is not; yet it appears to be an important link in the chain of causes. One must assume so from the frequency with which it is encountered. Hypertension provides an excellent example of what is probably true of many illnesses: a combination of varied factors conspire to bring them about. There are hereditary and familial influences, constitutional ones having to do with body form, chemical and physiological ones and, not the least important, psychological and sociological ones. Any purely unitary approach seems at present insufficient not only for understanding the illness but also for treating it. There is a tendency on the part of students of disease to root for the home team, so to speak, to see it only from their own point of view and not to look at the problem as a whole. A more philosophical attitude could lead to much needed co-operative studies.

Let me now give an example of one life history and point out those tendencies and patterns that are curiously characteristic of many sufferers from high blood pressure.

The patient I have in mind was a thirty-four-year-old married woman. During her early years she lived in Italy with her family under circumstances of hardship and great insecurity. Five of the seven children died in infancy. Only the patient and one brother, two years older, survived. When she was a child of four her mother died in childbirth. She could not remember her mother, but she appeared to have resented her death and to have had the feeling that had she lived she herself might have been healthy and happy instead of sickly and miserable.

After her mother's death she was brought up by her father and his old mother. Between her fourth and sixth years, however, she was separated from him because he had emigrated to the United States to prepare the way for the rest of the family. They followed—grandmother, brother and herself—when she was ten.

With the loss of his wife her father grew morose and irritable. Both he and her grandmother adopted a severe attitude toward the children. The old woman especially was harsh and forbidding, and the poor child received little affection and much discipline. In accordance with Italian tradition the boy of the family was allowed some liberty, but not she. To all this deprivation and discipline she reacted with extreme timidity and rigid obedience. She was full of fear and never dared to be defiant or rebellious, nor was she permitted to show anger. Instead she would become sulky at times, but more often she was secretly despondent and embittered. This pattern of behavior engendered in childhood persisted through her adolescent years, and indeed for the rest of her short life.

In her social behavior she was naturally greatly inhibited and constrained. She seldom left home and made few friends. Her closest companion was a girl of her own sort, timid and withdrawn. She avoided boys and never went through the "boy-crazy" stage. In later years she was nervous in the presence of men and always shunned them. Up to the time of her marriage she had had no sentimental or romantic encounters.

When she reached adulthood all these patterns of behavior established in childhood seemed to have remained with her. She was a docile young woman, full of fear and with a strong but unsatisfied need for dependence. At twenty-two she entered a marriage arranged for her by her prospective parents-in-law. Actually she married in defiance of her father's warning that the young man came from a family in which all the men were abusive toward their wives. She never loved her husband: her marriage was an unhappy one. Her husband turned out to be undependable, inconsiderate and harsh. He was given to outbursts of rage and sometimes beat her. Although she suffered from an endless series of humiliations at his hands she stayed with him and submitted to a life charged with bitterness. Perhaps her greatest crosses were the loss of her home, due to her husband's improvidence, and the feeling of degradation at the hands of her parents-in-law, with whom she and her two children were "forced to live as beggars." During this period of her life she became depressed, refused to eat, lost much weight and "looked like a corpse." All this suffering was in contrast to her previous romantic notions about marriage. She had hoped to find a quiet, peaceful person with whom she could live in contentment, but she found just the opposite. "I think my trouble started from the day I married," she said. "I might have had a tendency to high blood pressure but he aggravated it."

Many times she considered leaving her husband but always relented because of the children, on whom she gradually became increasingly dependent. She never quite gave up the hope of making her husband over into what she wanted him to be. The grievances she harbored against him were intense, but her fear was even greater, so that she was unable to express her resentment except by quarreling incessantly over money.

When she was about twenty-nine the emotional strain under which she lived reached a climax and it was at this time that her high blood pressure was first discovered. A number of circumstances conspired then to make her distress even more acute than before: continued impoverishment, pregnancy, her husband's cruelty and the sudden death of two people close to her. To all of these she reacted with extreme agitation, emotional outbursts, depression and obsessive fantasies of her own death. *Her lifelong tendency to suppress the expression of hostile feelings could not maintain itself in the face of so much inner turmoil.* She was filled with bitter hatred toward her husband. She wished him and his parents dead and was preoccupied with thoughts of destroying herself. She began to complain of headaches, palpitations, chilly sensations, fatigue and shortness of breath. By the time she was thirty-four her blood pressure was above 220 and it stayed at this high level until her death five years later. There were the usual changes in the heart and in the eyes, which are often, but by no means always, found in sufferers from arterial hypertension.

I have presented this somewhat long and unhappy chronicle not to try to prove a scientific point, which could hardly be achieved with one such history, but because though perhaps extreme in its poignant simplicity it is characteristic of many others.

The dynamics of more complicated and sophisticated personalities are naturally less transparent. Experience helps us to understand what goes on in the deeper, more obscure layers of the personality, even where the outer circumstances of a life are less manifestly tragic than they were in this one. The characteristic traits of personality common to most of these patients appear to be an excessive need for a secure, dependent relationship which, however, they are usually unable to find or to accept. Another characteristic is a weak, submissive attitude in which fear of injury, emotional isolation and suppression of hostility are prominent features. In addition there seems to be a tendency to experience frustration in relationships with other people, both social and sexual. Given this unstable emotional adaptation the applecart of their lives is easily upset. Frequently the balance is tipped by some event such as the loss of a member of the family or close friend or some other threat to the patient's feeling of safety. When such a threat occurs one usually sees a kind of acute emotional collapse; it is in this setting that the evidences of illness are liable to appear. Since the peculiar structure of the personality is present long before hypertension develops it seems justifiable to conclude that the high blood pressure itself does not account for the characteristic personality. More probably both the psychological disorder and the bodily disorder, which are observed, of course, by different methods, represent a basic failure in adaptation, often foreshadowed early in life and culminating eventually in this serious illness.

But what does all this mean to the patient and to his prospects for cure or relief? I have tried, in this book, always to come back to the patient himself and his needs and fears and hopes. Can anything be done to help him once he has developed high blood pressure, or to prevent its onset?

We have as yet no specific cure for this illness, though from the looks of things one cannot escape the feeling that the problem will "break" within the next few years.

In advanced cases the modern surgical approach is certainly warranted. It consists of a somewhat radical operation in which the chain of sympathetic nerves, lying along both sides of the spinal column, is removed. This procedure interrupts the nervous pathways along which pass impulses that result in constriction of the finer arterioles. When successful there may be a sustained fall in blood pressure. Sometimes the pressure mounts again after the lapse of several months but even when it does, the patient may not only feel much better but there may be a blessed relief from headache, and the damage to the eyes may disappear. Even though "cures" have been reported following operation it is fairly evident that such a procedure does not, in fact, deal directly with the cause of illness.

There can be little doubt that many patients have been greatly helped by judiciously applied psychotherapy, including advice as to rest and relaxation. Better still is teaching them to relax and helping them to deal, when possible, with their inner conflicts. Whether these can be successfully resolved even by prolonged and expert psychiatric treatment is hard to say. The decision as to the need and kind of psychotherapy must depend not upon the existence of a symptom such as high blood pressure but upon the personality of the sufferer and how he meets his problems.

A very striking instance of cure of hypertension by psychotherapy is reported in medical literature by Dr. Lewis B. Hill of Baltimore. It is noteworthy for many reasons, not only because of its apparently favorable outcome but also because of the clear view it gives us into the dynamics of the conflict.

The patient was a young man of thirty-two in whom hypertension had been known to exist for fourteen years. When he was eighteen his blood pressure was found to be $^{180}/_{120}$. At that time he had no symptoms of illness and with the exception of the elevated blood pressure, which was discovered in the course of a routine examination, a thorough investigation exposed no other evidence of disease. During the intervening fourteen years, blood-pressure readings were taken from time to time and fluctuated around $^{170}/_{110}$.

The young man carried a heavy hereditary load. All four grandparents had died in their sixties of diseases of the heart or blood vessels. Of their descendants, in the second generation six met similar deaths and two were living but suffering from hypertension. In his own generation not only he was afflicted but two cousins were also known to be. There may have been others. His own father was living and well at seventy with a normal blood pressure, as was his mother at sixty. He was described as active and athletic, unlike many hypertensives, and also as being of the plethoric type and pyknic physique—which means he was red faced and short and squat. This type is thought to be prone to develop high blood pressure. For hereditary and constitutional reasons, therefore, he might be looked upon as a good candidate for the disease from which he suffered.

What of the psychological reasons? The young man consulted Dr. Hill not because of his high blood pressure but because he had developed tension and anxiety in an acutely difficult situation, the nature of which is not divulged in the record. Dr. Hill states that: "Clinical cure resulted from brief therapy and the psychoanalysis was not completed." He then proceeds with this comment: "During one treatment hour the patient dramatized a scene which he dated as occurring after his eighth year. He appeared to lose consciousness and then built up a rage reaction at the height of which he grasped a weighted ash receiver and made a convincing attack upon my head with it, but actually avoided hitting me. His verbal offerings at this time were addressed to his mother and included mention of a G—— d—— buggy whip. As his rage increased he grew red in the face, with congested vessels in the neck. As the scene ended he was pallid and sweating." For a brief time thereafter he completely forgot the episode.

The patient then brought up the following memory: "As a child he had been teased by his sister till he struck her. His mother, as a punishment, took a pony whip with the evident intention of striking him. This was a very unusual thing, the whip merely happening to be at hand. In his fear he seized it from her hand, ran from her, and was brought to bay as he stood upon a bed, intending to hit her with it. He lost his courage, and as a final act of surrender with the hope of avoiding the whipping, meekly handed the whip to her. She struck him angrily. He had forgotten the experience completely till now.

"A short time after this analytic experience the blood pressure was reported $^{145}/_{90}$, and in the three years since then it has never read over $^{135}/_{90}$. Frequently it is $^{125}/_{85}$." Compare these figures with the ones given above which fluctuated about $^{170}/_{100}$. There was no other treatment which would affect blood pressure, and no change in his habits of living.

In discussing the facts Dr. Hill makes this comment: "I believe this patient experienced the whipping, that it was more painful and disruptive of self-confidence than he could tolerate," but Dr. Hill is not at all sure that the revenge scene actually occurred and that it was not a fantasy or, as he calls it, "a psychological truth." The reasons for this assumption rest on the argument that if the child had been able to defend himself or to attack or even to feel his rage effectively he would not have found necessary such a complete *repression* and *dissociation* of the episode from the rest of his personality. When a child is completely unable to react defensively to such a situation as this, all he can do is to repress it so that it retains almost no associational contact with the regular happenings of his life. A boy so defeated and defenseless is very likely to add a fantasy of revenge to the unhappy experience.

Here, then, is the psychological background of a case of hypertension. Who is to say whether it is more important or less than hereditary and constitutional influences? Are they not all contributory causes and should we not, in our treatment, direct our energies at the cause we can do most about removing? We cannot rewrite our pedigrees nor, by taking thought, add a cubit to our stature.

This extraordinary case fits in admirably with our present-day concept of the personality in hypertension. It exhibits the defenselessness of the child, the tendency to repress childhood memories, the suppression of rage, the mortal fear of destruction at the hands of a parent, the tendency to develop states of tension and anxiety. The only element missing is the one so frequently encountered in which an accident, a sudden death or illness, acts as a trigger mechanism. There may have been such in this patient, but it is not described. What is described is more important and much more difficult to unearth—that is, the early forgotten traumatic experience, in this instance the threat at the hands of the mother. Perhaps in each case some such forgotten experience lurks, only to be reactivated and rekindled later in life when the appropriate stimulus arises.

It is not improbable that such threatening and highly charged emotional experiences, though completely forgotten, repressed and dissociated from consciousness, still retain a kind of autonomous existence and that they find an outer expression through the more primitive part of the nervous apparatus—the so-called sympathetic or autonomic system. By the mediation of this system the repressed rage and fear can find bodily expression in one of many organs or organ systems. The choice of system involved—whether it be gastrointestinal, respiratory or, as in this case, vascular—and its ultimate breakdown may well depend upon hereditary and constitutional factors.

CHAPTER XII

The Cure and Control of Disease

CONSCIENTIOUS physicians eschew the word "cure." It is left to quacks to boast of their healing powers. This reticence and modesty have their historical background. The famous military surgeon Ambroise Paré, who was the first to abandon the practice of pouring boiling oil into gunshot wounds, set the pattern for us. "I dressed him and God healed him" was his dictum. That has remained the prevailing attitude of good doctors ever since. A bit of superstition undoubtedly clings to this sentiment. We keep our fingers crossed. We do not want to tempt the gods. Like the Chinese we revile our children at the temple gates for fear of bringing down the displeasure of evil spirits upon them. But the fact is we *can* cure some diseases.

The Rockefeller Institute for Medical Research was founded on the instigation of Mr. Frederic Gates, a retired Baptist minister who was engaged in helping the elder Rockefeller dispose of his fortune for philanthropic purposes. In June of 1897 Mr. Gates read Osler's *Principles and Practice of Medicine*, which was then and has remained to this day through fifteen revised editions the most widely read American medical textbook. The last three were edited by my former teacher Dr. Henry A. Christian, Hersey Professor of the Theory and Practice of Physic, Emeritus, at the Harvard Medical School—himself a pupil of Osler who, while greatly enlarging the text in keeping pace with the present tempo of medical progress, has at the same time continued its original tradition.

To his amazement Mr. Gates discovered that there was relatively scant attention paid to treatment. To put it in his own words:

> I found . . . that the best medical practice did not, and did not even pretend to, cure more than four or five diseases. . . . It was nature, and not the doctor . . . that performed the cures. . . . To the layman student like me, demanding cures and specifics, he [Osler] had no word of comfort whatever. In fact, I saw clearly from the work of this able and honest man that medicine had, with the few exceptions above mentioned, no cures, and that about all that medicine, up to 1897, could do was to nurse the patients and alleviate in some degree the suffering. . . .

In founding the Institute, the avowed purpose of which was to "cover the entire field of medical research in respect both to man and animals," Mr. Gates and his associates builded wisely. They did not set out to create an institute for the discovery of cures and specifics but rather to foster "the elements of high scientific achievement in medical research." Dr. Flexner, who had a major part in these important beginnings, tells the story of the founding of the Rockefeller Institute in the biography of Dr. William H. Welch.

Like happiness, a cure is seldom found by searching for it. Some cures are the logical outgrowth of deep scientific understanding, others are stumbled upon by accident and still others have grown out of the ancient experience and wisdom of the race. The movies give us the impression that a bearded scientist bending over his microscope in the small hours of the morning suddenly gives a shout and runs out on to the street—with his shirt on, to be sure—crying "Eureka! Eureka!" That is seldom if ever the history of a cure.

Perhaps only in the complicated field of chemotherapy have scientists succeeded in discovering cures that they set out to find. Paul Ehrlich's name (he of the "Silver Bullet") is inextricably linked to the miraculous science of chemotherapy. Man comes nearer impersonating the creator in this department of medical science than perhaps in any other. He prepares hitherto unknown chemical compounds, he changes their properties by the addition of new substances, he makes them dance to his tune. Finally after untold and costly labor he produces, if lucky, a compound that enters into chemical combination with an organism and vitiates its noxious influence. Such was the history of Ehrlich's Salvarsan, called "606" because that was its serial number in the list of chemical substances he had tried for the cure of syphilis. It has since been modified and replaced by neoarsphenamine. Such is the history of the revolutionary sulfa drugs: sulfanilamide, sulfapyridine, sulfathiazol, sulfadiazine and others, which often bring hope and life where before there were only despair and death. Such, too, is the history of atabrine for the prevention and cure of malaria; without this drug the jungle fighting of our marines would have been even more costly to life than it has been.

There are other substances of which the chemical composition is unknown or is discovered only after their usefulness in cruder form has been established. An example is the new drug penicillin, which has proved to be of such extraordinary value in the treatment of certain cases of infection with pus-producing bacteria. The story of its discovery is a fascinating one. In 1929 Alexander Fleming, an English bacteriologist, noticed that a familiar mold (Penicillium), similar to the one that grows on shoes at the seashore and on bread and cheese, had contaminated some of his culture media on which he was growing colonies of staphylococci. This is an ordinary enough occurrence in any bacteriological laboratory, usually resulting in a few curses and the discarding of the cultures. But Fleming observed that around a large colony of mold there was a clear area, the staphylococcic colonies having become transparent. This made him stop to think. Perhaps the mold produced some substance that killed the surrounding bacteria and thus accounted for the clear zone. He was right. It was no guess but a logical deduction based on a piece of very shrewd and careful observation. It earmarks him as a great scientist, for one of the criteria of greatness in science is the gift of learning from what appear to be mistakes. This has been the history of many important discoveries in medicine. It was not until 1940–42 that other English workers succeeded in purifying the product, analyzing it chemically, studying its properties, standardizing it and putting it to therapeutic use in ten selected cases of infection with staphylococcus and streptococcus. Since then their observations have been corroborated and extended by many scientific workers in this country, and the use of this new remedy is now established on firm ground.

The well-known relationship of iodine to the chemistry of the thyroid gland derives from the fact that a German chemist named Baumann noticed, some fifty years ago, a tiny purple fume rising from a heated extract of thyroid substance. He immediately recognized the fume as iodine in its gaseous form.

Sometimes cures or remedies grow out of a mistaken working hypothesis, but it is better to have a wrong one than none at all. When I was an intern, Dr. George R. Minot was one of our two resident physicians to whom we looked for advice and guidance. He was already interested in the treatment of pernicious anemia and experimented with various kinds of diets, believing, as has since been proved, that the anemia resulted from a faulty diet or an inability to assimilate certain elements of the diet. Later when he gave patients tumblerfuls of liver pulp to drink he was proceeding on the assumption that liver would stimulate the growth of new red blood corpuscles because it was known to have a growth-stimulating influence. Time and much labor have established pretty clearly that it was not the growth-stimulating influence that was important but the fact that liver supplies a missing dietary factor—proving that Minot's first "hunch" was correct. It was a fortunate one. Within a few years liver extract was chemically purified and standardized and reduced to a form that could be injected intramuscularly. The work that Minot and his associates did at the Harvard Medical School won them the Nobel prize. It was awarded jointly to him and to George H. Whipple of Rochester and to William P. Murphy of Boston who did the original work with Minot.

As you will have seen from the foregoing I have proceeded from the more rational approach to the problems of therapeutics represented by the science of chemotherapy, through discoveries made by taking felicitous advantage of accidents or mistakes, to "hunches" sometimes based on mistaken hypotheses. Many remedies have come to us in ways even more empirical. Some of these are recent, some ancient, and of many the rationale is far from clear. They are used for no better reason than that they seem to work. The discovery of heat treatment for syphilis of the brain, now administered either by deliberately giving the sufferers malaria or subjecting their bodies to various kinds of electrically generated heat waves, grew out of an observation of the Viennese neurologist Wagner-Jauregg, who noticed that these patients seemed to improve when they had a fever from some infection. One of our most useful drugs, digitalis, made from the leaf of the common foxglove, the familiar of many an herbaceous border, was discovered in 1785 by William Withering as one of twenty ingredients in an old wives' brew used for the treatment of dropsy.

There is a story that a certain pious Scottish physician, whose name I have forgotten, set out to find a remedy for rheumatics which plagued so many of his patients. Being a man of faith he believed that God would provide a remedy for every ailment in the very locality in which it occurred. That was his working hypothesis. Since rheumatism was most frequently found in damp, low-lying areas he looked there and found that the willow was the commonest tree. So he made a watery extract of willow bark. We know now that willow bark contains salicylic acid, which is the chemical basis of aspirin.

British seamen ate potato peels and drank lime juice to prevent scurvy long before vitamin C had been dreamed of. Quinine, of which the Japanese have had a monopoly since their invasion of the Dutch East Indies, was actually discovered not there but in Peru by Indians who found that the water of a certain lake cured them of chills and fever. Around its bank grew cinchona trees. Their shedding bark was extracted by the lake water which became thereby a decoction of quinine.

Of some of our common drugs the origins are certainly very ancient—drugs, for example, like mercury, ergot and morphine. Caffeine, or its closely related theobromine, in the form of coffee, tea or cocoa, is used by almost all peoples—as is alcohol. How the race has made these pharmacological discoveries we cannot say—perhaps by some trial and error method. People "feel better" after a good cup of tea. That some such method exists among untutored primitives whose native wisdom is not adulterated by knowledge we have reason to believe. I am not suggesting a Rousseauesque return of man to a state of nature but simply that a study of folklore medicine might yield us some valuable remedies. One of these recently culled from an ancient Chinese pharmacopeia is the new drug ephedrine.

Dr. Curt Richter of the Johns Hopkins Medical School, whose ingenious and important experiments on white rats I shall presently refer to, tells the story of a three-and-a-half-year-old boy who was admitted to the Johns Hopkins Hospital with a tumor of the adrenal gland—a fatal disease. The child had the habit of eating salt by the handful. He took to it as another child might to sugar or to jam. When he entered the hospital his salt-eating habit was stopped and he was put on the regular hospital diet. Unfortunately, he died soon thereafter. Now it appears that this child had discovered independently what it has taken experimental scientists many years to find out—that patients suffering from lesions of the adrenal glands are greatly benefited by the addition of large quantities of common salt to the diet.

Dr. Richter's white rats are also gifted scientists. He has shown that on a mixed standard diet of carbohydrates, proteins and fats, plus minerals and vitamins, the rats will maintain a predictable rate of growth and weight increase. Now if he offers his rats the ingredients of the diet unmixed they will still select just what they need to continue their growth and development at the usual rate. But even more remarkable is the fact that whereas a normal rat will consume relatively little salt a rat whose adrenal glands have been surgically removed will quickly and automatically increase its salt intake sufficiently to survive, whereas cagemates, similarly operated upon, will die when allowed only the normal salt ingredient in their diets. Rats deprived of their parathyroid glands will eat enough calcium to keep themselves alive and free from tetany. If the rats could consult medical literature they would find that calcium is given to babies with tetany as it is to adults whose parathyroid glands have been removed during an operation for goiter. Rats fed on thyroid extract develop a morbid appetite for weak solutions of iodine, the standard medicine given to patients whose thyroid glands are overactive.

There seems to be, therefore, some wisdom in the organism—some entelechy, as the Greeks had it—which leads it spontaneously to what is beneficial. No doubt civilized man who is guided by logic (that "systematic way of going wrong with confidence") has lost some of this talent. But there is perhaps more of it in us than we dare believe. Physicians of antiquity who extolled the *vis medicatrix naturae* may have had this in mind as well as rest, fresh air and sunshine. My teacher, Dr. Richard Cabot, used to speak half jokingly of "thalamo-therapy" —a fancy name he used for treatment by rest in bed. Much of our treatment is "nonspecific," as we say in medical jargon, and depends upon good nursing care, rest, good food, fresh air and a hopeful frame of mind. We try to put our patients in a situation in which nature can cure them of their ills.

With these preliminary remarks on cures and their discoveries I should like now to go on from where Mr. Gates left off forty-eight years ago in order to see what the status of medical treatment is now. For which diseases or illnesses have we specific remedies? For which is our treatment "general," "supportive," or "expectant"?

CHAPTER XIII

Recent Achievements and Tasks Ahead

PERHAPS for a moment we should cast another backward glance. In 1897 many of the medical commonplaces now known to almost every literate man had not even been dreamed of. There was no X-ray. There was no Wassermann test for syphilis. The spirochete that causes syphilis had not yet been discovered by Schaudinn. Vitamins were unheard of. There was no radium. Vaccination against typhoid fever had not been tried. In 1900 typhoid still occupied fourth place in the mortality list in the United States. In that year alone there were over thirty-five thousand deaths from it. During the Spanish-American War one of every five soldiers in our encampments was sick with typhoid. It is now such a rare disease that many of our recent medical graduates have never seen a case.

In 1897 no one had blood withdrawn from a vein for the purpose of making chemical or bacteriological studies. There were no such words as *allergy* or *basal metabolism*. The electrocardiogram had not been invented, nor had many other diagnostic procedures too numerous to catalogue.

Summer brought its heavy toll of deaths from infantile diarrhea. As it wore on toward early fall came typhoid fever. Diphtheria and scarlet fever arrived on winter's traces, often occurring in epidemics with a high death rate. I recall a huge gong in the hall of the Boston City Hospital which used, in earlier days, to be sounded at night when some child was choking to death from a diphtheritic membrane. The doctors would hurry to the patient to perform an intubation or sometimes a tracheotomy. Tetanus was a common and almost always lethal accompaniment of a serious wound. Cerebrospinal meningitis, then known as spotted fever, often raged in epidemics in which as many as 80 per cent of the victims died.

Today the summer diarrheas and typhoid fever have all but vanished. Diphtheria can be prevented by prophylactic inoculations of toxin-antitoxin mixtures or cured by antitoxic serum. Scarlet fever is now seldom a dangerous illness; its serious complications and consequences can be controlled by a specific serum and by the sulfa drugs. Tetanus is preventable. Cerebrospinal meningitis, rare except under the crowded conditions of cantonments, has in large measure lost its terrors, thanks again to sulfa drugs, though even before their use its disastrous effects had already been greatly mitigated after Flexner's introduction of serum treatment.

In one form or another the new sulfonamides appear to have a specific curative effect on many common bacterial diseases: pneumonia, gonorrhea, meningitis, puerperal fever, streptococcus and staphylococcus septicemia (called blood poisoning), and in various severe, sometimes fatal, local infections such as peritonitis, erysipelas and carbuncle. Using them to prevent hemolytic streptococcic infection can forestall the crippling damage to the heart which so often follows recurrent rheumatic fever. This chapter of medical history has just begun to be written. It promises to have a happy ending.

I do not, of course, mean to imply that everyone afflicted with these bacterial diseases can be cured of them. Much will depend upon the severity of the infection, the natural resistance of the individual, the promptness with which treatment is begun and the skill with which it is applied. But in the main we have found either the means to prevent this category of diseases or a rational, specific form of treatment, or both.

A few common bacterial infections have thus far defied the

quest for specific cures or preventive immunization. Chief among them is tuberculosis, called by Bunyan "captain of the men of death." (Osler used this same phrase of pneumonia. But the grim battery keeps changing officers; today it is led by diseases of the heart and arteries.) In the United States tuberculosis, therefore, no longer deserves this sinister characterization, having dropped as a cause of death from first place before 1900 to eighth in 1940. Known in its common pulmonary form as "consumption," it carried with it a death sentence and a life expectancy of not more than two years. How different the outlook today when early diagnosis and treatment in sanitaria and artificial collapse of the diseased lung make the future of the tuberculous patient a hopeful one! And in its other nonpulmonary forms, sunlight and surgery and general hygiene have accomplished equally encouraging results. No longer do we have to look into the wistfully reproachful eyes of the hunchback, whose spinal column buckled because of a tuberculous lesion of the vertebrae. He is now a rare sight. The death rate from tuberculosis, however, still remains enormous. In 1940 more than fifty thousand deaths occurred in this country.

Osler ends his chapter on tuberculosis with this apostrophe to the general practitioner:

> The leadership of the battle against this scourge is in your hands. Much has been done; much remains to do. By early diagnosis and prompt, systematic treatment of individual cases, by prompt recognition of contact cases, by striving in every possible way to improve the social condition of the poor, by joining actively in the work of the local and national antituberculosis societies you can help in the most important and the most hopeful campaign ever undertaken by the profession.

Improved social conditions, as well as isolation of cases, have undoubtedly contributed to the virtual disappearance of leprosy from this country. There are now probably not more than four hundred known cases in the United States, though it was estimated in 1937 that there were six to seven million lepers in the world. The few remaining ones here are gradually being discharged from leprosaria after prolonged treatment with injections of chaulmoogra oil.

Two other bacterial diseases of great historic importance must be mentioned: bubonic plague and typhus fever. For neither have we a specific cure; but we now know how they are transmitted, and from this knowledge has come the ability to prevent their spread.

After this cursory glance at bacterial diseases, let us next consider another category of infections—those due to the so-called filterable viruses. The list begins with the common cold and includes such familiars as influenza, measles (and its German cousin), mumps, chickenpox; also "shingles" or herpes. Certain others of a far more menacing character are infantile paralysis, encephalitis (known sometimes as sleeping sickness), yellow fever and rabies.

No specific cure has as yet been discovered for any of the virus diseases. But two of them, at least, are largely preventable: yellow fever, by destruction of the mosquitoes capable of transmitting it and by vaccination, and rabies, by muzzling and quarantining dogs and, of course, by the well-known Pasteur treatment. In 1897 the heroic American Commission on Yellow Fever made up of Walter Reed, Carroll, Lazear and Agramonte, under the direction of the army, had not yet demonstrated that yellow fever was transferred by the bite of a mosquito. Of Pasteur's prevention of rabies, Osler had this to say in 1897: "There is still much discussion as to the full value of this method, but if the protective inoculation can be successfully performed in dogs, there is no reason why the same should not hold good for man. . . ."

With the rapid growth of knowledge of the virus diseases we have reason to hope that prevention and specific treatment for others of them will come. Most welcome will this be in the case of infantile paralysis. The cause is known to be a filterable virus which can be transmitted to monkeys and to rats and mice. The infective agent is present in the brain and spinal cord, in the secretions of the nose, in feces and in the blood. Recently the virus has been found in sewage. The disease occurs sporadically and occasionally flares up in epidemic form. One attack confers immunity but as yet no artificial immunization has been possible. Nor are we entirely clear as to the means of transmission, though there is evidence that healthy carriers play an important part in spreading the disease, to which many are fortunately naturally resistant.

Infections may be due to bacteria which belong to the plant world, or to viruses (as yet unseen and unidentified, but known to be growing and living organisms), or to protozoa. Protozoa are single-celled animals of microscopic dimensions. The commonest and most important diseases caused by protozoa are syphilis, malaria, amoebic dysentery and trypanosomiasis, or African sleeping sickness.

If man's wisdom were as great as his knowledge, syphilis would cease to be a health problem. We know how to prevent it and how to cure it, but it is ubiquitous. The increasing frequency of its occurrence among adolescents is alarming. The ancient remedy, mercury, stemming from the time of Paracelsus, is still used, but the modern treatment dates from Ehrlich's famous discovery of Salvarsan in 1910. There is reason to believe that by the proper use of the newer arsenic preparations and of penicillin the infection can be entirely eradicated at the start.

"We do not yet know how the poison reaches the system," Osler wrote of malaria in 1897. Yet he held that

> the importance of the state of the soil in the etiology of malaria is universally recognized. It is seen particularly in low, marshy regions which have an abundant vegetable growth. . . . A tolerably high

temperature is one of the essential conditions for the development of the virus. . . . Many facts are on record which seem to indicate that the poison may be carried to some distance by winds. . . . That the distribution of the poison of malaria is influenced by gravity has long been conceded. Persons dwelling in the upper stories, or in buildings elevated some distance above the ground, are exempt to a marked degree.

As we read these extraordinarily shrewd observations it seems almost as if Osler were playing a game of blind man's buff with the mosquito.

That insect carriers could transmit disease had been first demonstrated in 1893 by Theobald Smith, one of the most illustrious figures in American medical history. His observations were made on Texas fever of cattle, a disease conveyed by the bite of ticks. Not until 1899 was Manson and Ross's discovery of the mosquito as the vector of malaria reported. The protozoan parasite in the blood had, however, been described in 1880 by Laveran, a French army surgeon; and quinine was and still is the best remedy for malaria.

Amoebic dysentery, while most frequent in the tropics, is common in temperate climates. Perhaps 5 to 10 per cent of the population in the United States is infected. Most of them are carriers; that is, they harbor the amoebae in their intestines without signs of illness. Any pollution of drinking water may therefore start an epidemic such as occurred in Chicago in 1933, when a cross connection between sewer pipes and water supply in a hotel resulted in many cases and deaths. We can anticipate a great increase in the number of carriers when our soldiers return from the tropics. It is fortunate that the hypodermic injection of the drug emetine usually stops the diarrhea promptly and that other new drugs, particularly diodoquin, are efficacious not only for prophylaxis but for ridding carriers of their amoebae.

African sleeping sickness is another important disease. It is caused by a microscopic, darting, corkscrewlike protozoan called the trypanosome which swarms in the blood stream of infected animals. The parasite may exist in frogs, fishes, birds, rats, horses, cattle, big game and men. Each species has its own kind of trypanosome, some disease-producing, others not. In equatorial Africa, in the so-called fly belts, sleeping sickness is rampant. One hundred thousand Negroes are said to have died of it in the Uganda in three years. The sickness is accompanied by extreme weakness, mental dullness, paralyses, convulsions, coma and death. It is the bite of the tsetse fly that introduces the trypanosomes into the bodies of men and animals. Neither the parasite nor the means of transmission was known before the beginning of this century. There are several remedial agents that are valuable for the treatment of African sleeping sickness. But eradication of this disease and prevention of its spread are a challenging and extremely difficult public-health problem, closely related to the economic future of equatorial Africa.

Not all the parasites that enter the body are of microscopic dimensions. Some tapeworms may reach a length of twenty-five to thirty feet. From the point of view of public health, however, it is the smaller worms that cause most damage, principally, of course, hookworms. Now recognized as widespread in the southern states, they were almost unknown before the beginning of this century. In 1901 seven cases were reported here. A year later the story was a different one: Stiles had shown that hookworm infection prevailed widely throughout the southern states and that it was the chief cause of the anemia and poor health so common in many districts. By 1916 it was recognized that the southern United States was badly infected: more than 12 per cent of cotton-mill employees and in various districts from 20 to 80 per cent of the population. In the meantime the mode of infection had been investigated and the extraordinary discovery made that the larvae of the worm usually enter the body through the skin of the feet. By a devious course through the human body, taking nearly seven weeks, they finally end up in the intestinal tract where they live in married bliss, the victim discharging as many as four million eggs in a single bowel movement. To rid a section of the population of its infestation—and of the anemia, apathy and malnutrition resulting from this parasitic disease—requires a campaign of sanitary education including the introduction of latrines or other means of sewage disposal and the wearing of shoes and stockings. In addition, in order to free infected persons of their worms it is necessary to treat them with one of several chemicals (carbon tetrachloride, known commercially as Carbona, is one of them). All this is new knowledge.

In his struggle for survival, man is exposed not only to bacteria, viruses, protozoa and other parasites but to many intoxicating substances as well. Some, such as lead and arsenic, he may encounter in his work. Although we have no specific cures for the diseases caused by these poisons, much has been done in the past few decades to improve conditions in industry and thereby to lessen the danger to workers. The recent autobiography of Dr. Alice Hamilton, *Exploring the Dangerous Trades,* tells the dramatic story of her pioneer work.

Food poisoning, popularly but incorrectly called "ptomaine poisoning," is far less common than it was, due to modern methods of processing, canning, refrigeration, handling and transportation. But poisoning by alcohol has been and remains one of the most important and perplexing problems that medicine has to face.

I refer, of course, to chronic alcoholism. It is described by Osler as "very difficult to treat, and once fully established, the habit rarely is abandoned." When medical science discovers how to prevent or cure chronic alcoholic addiction the world will be a happier place. Prohibition cannot solve this problem. Its magnitude may be inferred from these scant statistics: approximately 10 to 25 per cent of admissions to all mental hospitals in this country are the direct or remote result of overindulgence in liquor. For every such patient one can safely assume a background or setting of economic waste, failure, misery and despair, usually involving both himself and those close to him. Psychiatrists are gradually gaining some insight into the personality of the drunkard. They recognize that indulgence is often a symptom of a severe disturbance of the personality. It must be honestly stated that our knowledge is still too imperfect for us to have a great deal to contribute except general hygiene, correction of dietary deficiencies and custodial care. In some cases psychotherapy may be of help, and self-treatment in groups through such organizations as Alcoholics Anonymous often holds out the best hope.

Not only what men put into their mouths steals away their brains—sometimes it is what they do not put in. Pellagra, a disease in which the roughening and redness of the exposed parts of the skin are often an early sign, may be accompanied by mental confusion, depression, change in disposition and even by hallucinations. In Osler's second edition it was listed under "The Intoxications." Pellagra was then believed to be the result of eating spoiled corn. It has since been shown to be a deficiency disease, "resulting from a lack of necessary ingredients in the diet, especially too little proteins and fresh vegetables but also too much carbohydrate." Lack of vitamin B_2 undoubtedly plays a most important role in pellagra as it does in many of the symptoms of chronic alcoholism.

The whole category of deficiency diseases and their cure by vitamins is new knowledge. The word vitamin was not coined until 1912.

The list of deficiency diseases includes (besides pellagra) beriberi, scurvy, night blindness, rickets, sprue and several others less commonly known. None of these was truly recognized as such in 1897 and the cures and preventives were empirical ones. Even then, however, the Board of Trade required that a sufficient supply of antiscorbutic (against scurvy) articles of diet such as lemon juice and fresh vegetables be taken on each ship. Scurvy, once "the plague of mariners," has become rare.

Deficiency diseases are not always caused by inadequate diet. There are, undoubtedly, some circumstances in which though the supply of materials is ample, their utilization is for some reason or other impeded. There are others in which the body does not manufacture a sufficient supply of an essential chemical substance. Sometimes, on the other hand, the supply may be overabundant and the result equally harmful. I have in mind particularly the derangements of the glands of internal secretion. These, too, both as to recognition and modes of treatment, form a new, important and rapidly growing department of medicine. Whereas Osler originally described only disturbances of the adrenals and the thyroid gland, today we have valuable information about several others, especially the pituitary and sex glands. The application of physiological and chemical methods and modern surgical techniques has vastly extended our knowledge of these extraordinary, vital structures. In almost no other branch of medical research have more brilliant discoveries been made. A kind of chemistry of the personality is being developed, and more and more the reciprocal relationship between the mind and the body is being exemplified in this field.

Other diseases to which chemical knowledge has brought new and valuable insight are such disturbances of metabolism as gout, diabetes, obesity and acidosis, and the various disorders of the blood-forming organs known as the anemias. I have already alluded to the successful treatment of pernicious anemia by the injection of purified liver extracts.

In fifty years medicine has made conspicuous progress in dealing successfully with a variety of diseases: bacterial, protozoal, parasitic and intoxicating; diseases due to dietary deficiencies and to disturbances of glandular secretions and metabolism. What then remains? What of the so-called degenerative diseases? What of sudden death from "heart attacks"; what of strokes and apoplexy? What of arteriosclerosis; what of the obscure and tragic derangements of the central nervous system; what of cancer which hangs over so many like a sword, and what of the "insanities," perhaps more devastating than any of the others?

If Mr. Gates were alive today he might again be dismayed were he to turn to that part only of Osler's textbook which treats of these subjects. For we have as yet no specific cures or sure preventives. What Osler said in 1897 of arteriosclerosis is, to the best of our knowledge, true today:

> As an involution process arteriosclerosis is an accompaniment of old age, and is the expression of the natural wear and tear to which the tubes are subjected. Longevity is a vascular question, and has been well expressed in the axiom "that a man is only as old as his arteries." To a majority of men death comes primarily or secondarily through this portal. The onset of what may be called physiological arteriosclerosis depends, in the first place, upon the quality of arterial tissue (vital rubber) which the individual has inherited, and secondly upon the amount of wear and tear to which he has subjected it. That the former plays the most important *rôle* is shown in the cases in which arteriosclerosis sets in early in life in individuals in whom none of the recognized etiological [causative] factors can be found. Thus, for instance, a man of twenty-eight or twenty-nine may have arteries of a man of sixty, and a man of forty may present vessels as much degenerated as they should be at eighty. Entire families sometimes show this tendency to early arteriosclerosis—a tendency which cannot be explained in any other way than that in the make-up of the machine bad material was used for the tubing.

These wise remarks could hardly be improved upon today, perhaps, however, heightened by Dr. Peyton Rous of the Rockefeller Institute, with his comment: "The accustomed responses of our own bodies have resisted modernization . . . . senility has the right of way."

Though our treatment of such conditions, as for example

angina pectoris, is based upon more accurate knowledge of the blood supply to the heart muscle; and though we have refined our diagnostic methods, we cannot provide new hearts for old, nor even new blood vessels. Nor can we as yet delay the aging process or add to man's allotted years. It is not too much to believe that even this domain may open up its secrets to man's inquiring mind and that another fifty years may deliver up the answer to many baffling questions. How the face and figure of our world will look when we all achieve biblical ages I cannot predict, nor whether we shall count that day a blessing.

In the battle with cancer much has been accomplished, though the cause still remains obscure. Through an active campaign of education of the profession and the laity, by more prompt diagnosis, by the use of radium, X-ray and surgery many lives have been saved and much suffering averted.

Since our guidebook in this sight-seeing tour has been a textbook of medicine, I have, up to now, said little of surgery. The technical advances since the turn of the century have been fabulous: rubber gloves, new suture materials, improved asepsis and anesthesia, methods of treating shock and of avoiding such complications as paralysis of the intestines and collapse of the lung. And new territories have been opened up by pioneers in chest surgery and brain surgery.

For many years it has been my custom to accompany into the operating room each one of my patients who has required a major operation. If possible, I try to see him before anesthesia is induced and as he comes out. Patients vary greatly in their response to this ordeal—from frank fear to stoicism and bravado. And the surgeons vary as much. There are slapdash ones and meticulous ones, peppery, temperamental ones and phlegmatic ones. As I stand by, becapped and begowned, trying to keep out of the way, I am always struck with the beauty of the scene, so greatly enhanced by the gray-green walls that have replaced glazed-white bathroom tile, and I am impressed with the wonderful adaptation to purpose of hand and instrument. Man has surely achieved great heights of order, co-ordination and control in this uniquely co-operative effort in which so many play their part—surgeon, assistants, nurses, orderlies, hospital administrator, engineer, instrument maker, drug manufacturer and sometimes even the poor patient.

Two years ago a woman of sixty consulted me because of severe insomnia. She was kept awake by the sour contents of her stomach coming up into her gullet and burning her throat. To reduce the acidity of her gastric juice she had the habit of drinking milk or eating a cracker about every hour and taking frequent doses of alkaline powders. She was fast becoming more and more "neurotic" and lived only for the short intervals in which she was free from discomfort. Her conversation dealt principally with her stomach and its contents. It turned out that she had a hernia of the diaphragm; that is, an opening in the diaphragm through which part of her stomach protruded from the abdomen up into the cavity of her chest. At the point where it passed through the opening in the diaphragm the stomach was constricted in hourglass fashion. Before long this unfortunate woman began to vomit incessantly and to lose weight. A series of X-ray studies showed progressive changes until finally her stomach not only lay almost wholly in her chest, but was folded over on itself. Both her age and the serious nature of her illness made the outlook for operative interference none too hopeful, and yet there was no other chance for her recovery—indeed, for her survival. The operation was a stormy one. To grapple with an elusive stomach and haul it into place, to close the gap in the diaphragm, to remove bands of adhesions and return the stomach to its natural abode make a difficult and tricky procedure. Such manipulation of the viscera produces a condition of shock, especially when one side of the chest cavity is opened and the lung ceases to expand. The patient showed all evidence of shock: ashen pallor, clammy skin, thready pulse, low blood pressure.

During the operation she inhaled a great deal of mucous secretion. The stage was set for a postoperative pneumonia. I was greatly impressed with the varied procedures employed to avert calamity. While she was still in the operating room she was given a blood transfusion and also an intravenous injection of a solution of glucose containing sulfadiazine. Powdered sulfanilamide was sprinkled inside her abdominal cavity and one drainage tube was inserted under the diaphragm and allowed to protrude through the closed skin wound, in case of peritoneal infection. Then a specialist was sent for to insert a long tubular bronchoscope into her lungs through which all the inhaled material was sucked out by a mechanical apparatus. The patient was next allowed to breathe a mixture of oxygen and carbon dioxide which served not only to restore the normal oxygen content to her blood and tissues but also, by stimulating deep breathing, enabled her to blow off the ether vapor and expand her partially collapsed lung. A few months later she was playing golf and enjoying her victuals. A decade or so earlier, she would have died.

And yet one should not be too awed or bewildered by modern surgery. Harvey Cushing, who was responsible for so many of these technical advances, used to argue that there was no difference between medicine and surgery. What he meant was that in spite of their unlike historical origins, they now rested on the same intellectual substratum, on the same careful observations, the same logical inferences. The success of each depends upon accurate and early diagnosis. This great master of surgery had the habit of belittling the surgeon's skill, calling it "mere carpentry." He was wise enough to know that even his rare talent could not have borne fruit without the contributions that internal medicine, physiology and pathology have brought to bear on the problems that daily confronted him and to which he himself added so much of lasting value.

The diminishing death rate from appendicitis has resulted largely from early diagnosis by medical men, although it is the surgeons who have taught us its potential danger. In the first edition of Osler's *Textbook* (1892) he says that the medical treatment of appendicitis can be expressed in three words—rest, opium and enemas(!) Almost every intelligent layman now knows how mistaken he was. He corrected himself three years later with this terse remark: "There is no medical treatment of appendicitis." The same sentence is repeated in the latest edition, after nearly fifty years.

To turn now from the concreteness of surgery to psychiatry: In 1897 Osler mentions briefly, under Diseases of the Nervous System, hysteria, neurasthenia and the traumatic neuroses and dwells particularly on the Weir Mitchell method of treatment, so popular in the nineties, which consisted of isolation, rest, diet, massage and electricity. Freud's great work was then just at its beginning. His studies had not yet influenced medical thought as they have during the past few decades. The importance of anxiety and repression was not yet understood nor the effects of the emotions on bodily functions. Psychoanalysis had hardly been heard of in this country. The mental hygiene movement had not been initiated, nor child guidance. Our mental hospitals were still "insane asylums." Occupational therapy was undeveloped (as in many respects it still is); "shock" treatment, recently come into such prominence, was unknown. Psychosomatic medicine, which I have discussed in previous chapters, was unheralded and unsung. Psychiatry and medicine were farther apart then than they were in antiquity and much farther than they are today. Their approximation is one of the most important steps, as yet perhaps not fully appreciated, which modern medicine has taken.

I have tried in this chapter to indicate some of the goals that medicine has achieved during the last half century in the direction of the cure and control of illness and disease. Who can say whether the next fifty years will yield as much? Physicians and other men of science so often proudly disclaim any interest in philosophy or knowledge of it. There need be no quarrel between natural science and philosophy. A deeper understanding of man's values, his social institutions and ethical concepts may prove them to be more closely related to his illness and health than we have dared believe.

CHAPTER XIV

Convalescence and Chronic Disease

SOME fifteen or twenty years ago a member of the staff of the Bellevue Hospital in New York modeled a statue which he called "Discharged—Cured." It represented a patient leaving the hospital after a mastoid operation. He had been ill for several weeks. His clothes hung loosely on him, the muscles wasted, the face gaunt, the eyes deep set with a frightened, hopeless look in them. How little imagination it takes to follow this man out through the revolving hospital door into the bewildering and noisy city—a little trembly, pallid and sweaty, short of breath, irritable, worried and unsure. Cured indeed!

By the time their patients begin to convalesce many doctors are a bit bored and would rather turn to the challenge of a "red-hot appendix" or "a good sick pneumonia." Convalescence, they think, is a job to be supervised by trained nurses or by a soft-spoken, hand-holding fellow with a good bedside manner or, if it concerns a hospital patient, by the Social Service Department.

We know all too little about the convalescent state and how to facilitate and expedite it. In 1939 a Conference on Convalescent Care was held at the New York Academy of Medicine under the auspices of its Committee on Public Health Relations. There were many distinguished speakers. As I listened to them and perused the report of the conference I was struck not only with the frank confession of ignorance about many aspects of convalescent care but also, and more so, with the wholly inadequate provisions we have for it. We have chosen to meet the problem almost as if it did not exist.

For example, one speaker—an authority in the field of heart disease—stated that at a conservative estimate, diseases of the heart affected about 2 per cent of the population. In other words, if this estimate is correct, there are approximately 2,500,000 cardiac invalids in the United States. Many of them require more or less prolonged rest in bed, and yet there are fewer than a thousand beds available. Almost half of these beds are in New York State and of the total number 75 per cent are restricted to the care of children.

In New York City there are 58 convalescent homes with a total bed capacity of 4,040. All are maintained by voluntary effort, although the taxpayers contribute a paltry $350,000 annually toward the maintenance of certain needy convalescent patients. Admission to these homes is none too easy to obtain. There are many rules and restrictions, and a good deal of shopping around is necessary just when the patient is most enfeebled, discouraged and frightened. If you happen to be colored instead of white there is almost no place to convalesce except in your own "cold-water-walk-up." But of these subjects I shall speak later.

There was much discussion at the conference of the "psychological aspects of convalescence." Indeed one speaker stated that our ignorance of convalescent care was partly due to *over-emphasis* of this very subject. I cannot agree with him, nor with those others who look upon convalescence as though it concerned *either* the body or else the mind. Is there not some confusion here based on a prevailing tendency to think in "either-or" terms? From my own experience I should be willing to make the statement that every convalescent patient presents both physical and psychological problems. Of course the two are interrelated. Have you ever encountered a mind without a body or (except in politics) a body without a mind? Because we emphasize one point of view, need we derogate the other?

Professor Carl Becker, in his book *The Heavenly City of the Eighteenth Century Philosophers,* says:

> . . . because the modern mind has a predilection for looking at men and things in this way [the historical-scientific], it finds a high degree of mental satisfaction in doing it; and mental satisfaction is always worthwhile, for the simple reason that when the mind is satisfied with the pattern of things it sees, it has what it calls an "explanation" of the things—it has found the "cause" of them.

Now the medical mind is, of course, steeped in this modern tradition. Its ardor in establishing "causes" no doubt yields great satisfaction—sometimes, however, at the cost of truth. In medical jargon the "cause" of a disease is spoken of as its etiology. Etiology actually is the word for the science of the study of causes and should not be used interchangeably with the word cause. The study of causes leads quickly into the realm of metaphysics. From antiquity the nature of "causality" has occupied the attention of philosophers. Modern physicists are more self-critical in this regard and have carefully defined and examined the premises of their thought. Not so, modern physicians, who tend toward a certain practical naïveté in these fundamental matters. If a man swallows a culture of typhoid bacilli and "comes down" with the disease then it is clear that the bacilli "caused" the disease. But if another man develops a swelling in his neck, bulging eyeballs, rapid heart rate, sweating, loss of weight and irritability, we can, to be sure, ascribe his illness to an increased secretion of thyroxin, but when we ask why his thyroid gland is working overtime we may find ourselves deeply involved, not only in his sympathetic nervous system but mayhap in his heredity, his job, his marriage, his religious convictions, his ambitions, achievements, aggressions and frustrations. All may have important "etiological" bearing on his illness. No single one of them is necessarily the cause.

And so in the reverse process—in the return to health from illness one always deals with multiple causes. It is part of the doctor's job to set the reverse process in motion, or at least not to interfere with its orderly progress. Man has discovered for himself some of the circumstances that help to restore him to health: rest, quiet, proper attention to diet and nutrition, friendly sympathetic faces, the ministrations of gentle hands, flowers, books and various little attentions. All these win him back to life, gratify the need for love and care which his illness has magnified, and gradually permit him to abandon the complete self-absorption which invalidism has demanded of him and to turn again toward others and toward the world of objects around him. In the proper timing and encouragement of this process lies the art of convalescent care.

Here, as in other departments of civilian medicine, much will be learned from the experiences of the war. Our army air force, for example, has instituted an intelligent and active program directed toward the problems of convalescence. Something has been done about the endless days of boredom in which the convalescent soldier hung around the hospital ward in his dingy bathrobe. An active plan of rehabilitation is begun early and carried on until the man is returned to his unit or transferred elsewhere. It includes reconditioning, calisthenics, vocational training and even the study of foreign languages. In the army air force, according to Brigadier General David Grant, the average period of convalescence from pneumonia has been cut down from forty-eight days to thirty-one.

All this was a new departure for the army. Heretofore a soldier was considered either sick or well. When he was sick he was in a hospital, when well he was returned to duty. Although this attitude fitted in better with army routine and "paper work" it did not make for an efficient force. Many remained too long in the wards, growing soft and demoralized from idleness, and others were required to undergo hardships and exposure for which they were not yet fit.

We should profit by these military experiences. In civil practice, when a man is up and about he usually considers himself ready for work. Laborers, office workers and overburdened housewives return to their duties, in most instances, before they are ready to. A few days' recuperation after the flu may not only avert a recurrence but also prevent weeks of exhaustion and depression. After childbirth or a major operation or any serious illness this is obviously even more true.

If you stop to think a moment you will realize that before very long a large proportion of the population of the world will be made up of convalescents or chronic invalids. Even in this country, where civilians have not been directly damaged by the war, with eleven million men under arms and with fighting going on on eighty-two major fronts, the number of casualties is sure to be high. Up to March, 1944, the total number discharged because of disabilities was over two hundred thousand, and nearly thirty thousand discharges a month occurred because of nervous and mental illnesses alone. In addition, provision had to be made for many cases of tuberculosis, of malaria, of amoebic dysentery and, of course, for general medical and surgical disorders. Some three hundred thousand beds to care for the hospitalized neuropsychiatric cases alone have been estimated as necessary.

Since the passage of the Barden-LaFollette Bill, establishing Federal Rehabilitation Services under the Federal Security Administration, the authority has been created for a nation-wide rehabilitation program. There is great danger, however, that the ex-soldiers will fall between the many groups who have staked out claims to help them. The problems facing discharged service men are many and perplexing, especially for those released because of nervous and mental disabilities and also for those rejected from the draft for the same reason. As Dr. Thomas Rennie puts it:

Socially these men find the adjustment at home difficult. They belong to no recognized group and in many places there are no organized resources for appropriate recreation. Companionship is denied them because their contemporaries are in service. Unable to work or too embarrassed to seek for work, many of them stay at home, occasionally wandering out in the evening alone to a movie—ashamed to telephone former friends, uncertain as to how to explain their reappearance into civilian life, fabricating some physical symptom to explain their discharge. Many of these men know their diagnoses. Their attempts to read up on the subject of psychoneurosis confuses them. Parents are equally baffled and their apprehensiveness, fear and oversolicitude make the problem worse. Well-meaning friends sometimes add the final damage by suggesting that the soldier is entitled to compensation and should become a ward of the government. The man flounders for months while the Veterans' Administration adjudicates his claim.

A beginning has been made in an effort to solve these problems—but only a beginning. A number of rehabilitation clinics already exist. There will be need for many more—well staffed with psychiatrists and properly trained social workers. The task must be co-ordinated with a vocational retraining and re-employment program. This work should be paid for by the federal government. After demobilization many doctors now in the service could be employed on a part-time basis to help in the task of rehabilitation. Much of value to civilian medicine has undoubtedly been learned, especially in the direction of shorter psychotherapeutic procedures and of occupational therapy, which has fortunately begun to move beyond the stage of weaving baskets and hammering out pewter ashtrays.

But to return to civil practice: When convalescence is prolonged many new problems may arise that will require careful supervision and management. A cranky, self-centered, petulant invalid can upset a whole family, and so can a saintly, long-suffering, patient one. It is perhaps worth remembering that many convalescents exhibit evidence of mental depression. They may be oversensitive, excessively dependent and introspective, slowed up in their mental processes, and they may experience difficulty in accomplishing the simplest tasks. I have so often seen convalescents burst into tears when anyone dear to them entered the room. With increased physical strength and with the return of normal appetite and sleep these symptoms usually vanish, but it is important for the doctor to direct his attention to the mental depression and to help the family in their dealings with their sick relative.

If one needs tact and resourcefulness and expert medical knowledge to give convalescent care, rare wisdom and almost a kind of heroism may be called for to treat the chronic invalid and the hopelessly sick. To sit by and see a man slip into progressive enfeeblement, suffering and the dashing of his hopes is a painful experience for a doctor. If he is himself a person of wisdom and courage he may be a pillar of strength and a source of hope and comfort. Great attention to detail may save his bed-ridden patient much discomfort and suffering. It is the doctor's job to help his patient accept the restrictions and limitations which invalidism imposes on him and to direct his remaining energies toward satisfying goals. Sometimes the doctor must descend with his patient almost into the valley of the shadow. Many of our patients who know they are going to die would be comforted by talking freely with us about their fate, but this requires a self-possession and integrity of spirit which we cannot often lay claim to.

I suspect that to die well one must have lived well. Like other doctors I have witnessed extraordinary reactions to impending death—craven fear and anger, sublime peace and even transcendent physical beauty.

Although western man has become skillful and expert at killing he has given relatively little thought to dying. He trots out his religion like the hired palms of the undertaker's parlor when the need arises. He lives his life unprepared to die. He is gripped by intense and agonizing fear when confronted by the frightfulness of death. Perhaps this primitive attitude reflects a fault in our spiritual education.

I have never been an enthusiast for euthanasia, because in my experience very few sufferers really want to die. It is those who watch them suffer who want them to, because they cannot endure the distressing spectacle. They cannot admit to consciousness their own wish for relief and therefore assume that it is the patient who wants to die. The sick man himself usually seeks only reprieve from his suffering and lives for the next moment of surcease and for the small things that make up his day: the rearrangement of his pillows, a cool drink, a shot of morphine. It is the doctor's job to conserve life, not to destroy it. If society determines to end suffering then the doctor should be called upon to give his expert opinion on the probable course of the illness and perhaps to administer the *coup de grâce,* but he should have no part in deciding who should live and who should die. Of all suffering perhaps the mental anguish and feeling of guilt of a severe depression are the worst. And yet I have never heard anyone suggest that these sufferers be mercifully dispatched.

Chronic invalids may sometimes achieve good lives in spite of severe hardships and handicaps. Who is to say that they would be "better off dead"? Without some whom I have known, the world would be a poorer place.

Yet the problem of chronic illness is staggering in its dimensions and one too seldom considered from a public-health point of view. It is estimated, for example, that in the United States about twenty-three million persons suffer from some form of chronic disease. As causes of death these diseases are, in order of importance: affections of the heart, cancer, arteriosclerosis and high blood pressure. As causes of disability, however, nervous and mental disorders head the list, followed by rheumatism and heart diseases, and then tuberculosis, arteriosclerosis and high blood pressure.

Seventy years ago these chronic diseases caused only one-fifteenth of all deaths; today they are responsible for as many as one-half. At first glance one might be led to suppose that there had been an enormous increase in their occurrence, that the wear and tear of modern industrial life were responsible for the greater number of deaths now attributable to these causes. But such an interpretation of facts would be erroneous. It appears that those of us who escape the fatal illnesses of childhood and early life—now so largely preventable—survive to middle life and old age, only to succumb eventually to the degenerative diseases attendant upon these later periods. According to statistics gathered by the Metropolitan Life Insurance Company, a child born in 1901 had an average life expectancy of forty-nine years, whereas for one born in 1937 the expectancy has increased to over sixty-one years. As Boas puts it: "Although the pestilences have been brought under control, the great volume of chronic diseases form a plague of as great proportion as any to which mankind has been subject." A hidden and insidious plague, he calls it, lacking the dramatic qualities of a major epidemic but all the more deadly because its ravages are not recognized. Its consequences are not only illness and death but destitution and disruption of family life.

Dr. Boas has provided us with much valuable statistical material in his book *The Unseen Plague—Chronic Disease*. For example, "two out of every hundred persons in the United States have a permanent orthopedic impairment of such a serious nature that they are partially or completely crippled, deformed or paralyzed." Of two million six hundred thousand with such disabilities more than five hundred thousand are incapacitated. There are nearly seven million sufferers from rheumatism and nearly four million from diseases of the heart and about one and a half million afflicted with chronic severe nervous and mental disorders requiring hospitalization. The annual admission rate to mental hospitals is at least seventy-five thousand. This means that, on the average, no fewer than two hundred persons are admitted to mental hospitals on each and every day of the year. The number of neuropsychiatric disorders that exist in the population at large can be roughly estimated from the shockingly high rate of rejections from the draft for this cause alone.

"The matrix of medicine," as Dr. Alan Gregg of the Rockefeller Foundation calls it, has changed in the last decades and accordingly, in large measure, the doctor's job. More and more the acutely ill, both physically and mentally, are treated in hospitals, and more and more the practitioner of medicine aims at the prevention and the amelioration of chronic diseases, even when he cannot cure them.

CHAPTER XV

The Prevention of Illness

FROM what has gone before you will have understood that there is a public medicine and a private medicine; the one is concerned with problems of sanitation and the prevention of epidemic disease, with nutrition and the feeding of populations, the other with sick individuals and their restoration to health. The distinction is, to be sure, somewhat academic, somewhat specious. A sick man—one incapacitated for work—may become a public charge who no longer pulls his weight in the community. His wife and children suffer and, in a sense, we all do. It may sound sentimental to say that a Vermont farmer who complains of "cold stummick" and who can no longer relish his pie for breakfast is our concern. But he is, not because we need accept the burden of being our brother's keeper but because in ever widening circles his illness will affect the security and prospects for education of his children, the milk production of his herd, his own purchasing power, not to mention such imponderables as his peace of mind and contentment. Whether he is our near neighbor or lives beyond the mountains he still is our concern. Now if one multiplies the Vermont farmer by many millions who suffer from ordinary complaints—headache, constipation, backache, lumbago, fatigue, palpitations, chronic cough, sleeplessness—it becomes fairly clear that the minor ailments of man may become social health problems of the first magnitude. Many serious and perhaps fatal illnesses such as cancer, syphilis, tuberculosis, diabetes and hypertension announce themselves by just such "minor" symptoms. I recall once asking a young colored man what his mother had died of. He replied: "Ah don't know, Boss; hit wahn't nothin' serious"! Humorous though it sounds there is more in his remark than at first strikes the ear. What he meant was that she had suffered from a slight indisposition which turned into an illness from which she eventually died.

In the care of mental and emotional disorders *prevention* is especially important. These illnesses are costly in time and money. They cause intense suffering not only to the patient himself but to those close to him as well. Once they have become chronic the prognosis is so often "guarded"—the word with which medical cant tempers the wind of unacknowledged pessimism. Many of these disorders are, to be sure, difficult—perhaps impossible—to prevent, but not all of them. It is now recognized that the best time to forestall what are called maladjustments is in childhood and adolescence when storm warnings are too often ignored.

The distinction between public and private medicine cannot be sharply drawn. No practitioner of medicine whose concern is with the health and welfare of individuals need feel inferior to the sanitarian or even to the scientist whose discoveries can affect the welfare of millions. What matters is how seriously he takes his job. Whether he recognizes it or not the practice of medicine is a public service. It is not a work to be approached with the attitude of a smalltime shopkeeper who hands notions over the counter in exchange for a dollar bill.

If medical practice is to fulfill its most important function—the prevention and early detection of physical and mental illness—then several conditions must be met. First, a sufficient supply of well-trained doctors is needed. This is self-evident. Second, there must be no hindrance to bar the doctor from those who might wish to consult him. And third, there must be available, both to the doctor and to his patients, modern diagnostic facilities at a cost not too great.

Let me take up separately these three conditions that are necessary for the prevention of illness even though I have not included among them—perhaps the most important of all—the raising of the educational level of the community and the standard of living. Of a fairly large number of diseases it can be said that their incidence varies inversely with income level. For example, rheumatic fever, tuberculosis, nutritional disturbances occur far more frequently among the poor than among the comfortable, as do also accidents and injuries. In addition, syphilis and gonorrhea are the accompaniment of ignorance and carelessness and drunkenness.

As to the supply of doctors: It is usually estimated that for a civilian community in peacetime one doctor to approximately eight hundred population is the proper distribution. Doctors, however, are not all created free and equal. Some are good for one thing and some for another. In our large cities there are usually enough well-trained medical men to meet the needs, but this is much less true of sparsely settled rural communities. Even when there are enough doctors there may still be too great a lag between the time of "feeling sick" and the time of consulting a doctor. Several reasons exist for this which might be worth analyzing. Three principal ones occur to me: ignorance, fear and expense.

In spite of movies, lectures and popular books, baby clinics and health centers, the average layman is profoundly ignorant of the simplest facts of human physiology and hygiene. He is suggestible, to say the least, to clichés, old wives' tales and superstitions. He believes, for example, in "feeding a cold and starving a fever." He believes, of course, under almost any circumstances, in "a good cleaning out" of his intestinal tract. If he has a pain in his back or has to urinate frequently he believes that he must have "caught a cold" in his kidneys. If he is tired, irritable and sleepless he usually attributes the condition to "overwork," not realizing that overwork is more often a result of emotional disturbance than a cause of it. He treats his "acid condition"—whatever that is—with bicarbonate and expects vitamins to prevent colds and increase his energy. If he is fat he thinks he needs "a little thyroid." If he is thin he needs vitamins. If he has a skin eruption he irritates it by putting iodine on it. And so it goes and I must stress here that the indiscriminate use of over-advertised nostrums without proper medical advice can lead to most unfortunate results.

Unlike Dr. Richter's white rats which I mentioned previously, the average layman does not depend on trial and error or on empirical methods that make him feel better. Instead, he resorts to inadequate measures based on false theories and half knowledge. He is, of course, profoundly influenced by the daily barrage of radio plugs to which he exposes himself and by the car cards that force themselves on the jaded straphanger's attention.

During the period of lag between feeling sick and consulting a doctor there is frequently an attempt to forestall the evil day by self-administered home treatment. The evil, of course, is to call the doctor or to call on him. That is an admission of illness. It opens the door through which fear enters.

It is said that when Henry of Navarre rode into battle on his plumed charger, he exclaimed: "*Carcasse, tu trembles, mais si tu savais où je t'amène, tu tremblerais vraiment!*" (Body, you tremble, but if you knew whither I was leading you, you would tremble indeed!) I am constantly struck by the fear and trembling with which even educated and sophisticated people consult their doctors. Their smattering of medical knowledge is just enough so that a slight needle scratch of pain or discomfort passes through the amplifying system of their anxiety to emerge as a roar and a din. Such patients, if they are not excessively hypochondriacal, can be enormously relieved by a careful and painstaking examination. If there is any pooh-poohing to be done it must be done after the examination. It is the custom of many excellent doctors to send their patients a complete transcript of all the facts found on physical examination. I doubt the wisdom or usefulness of such a procedure. In the first place no layman can evaluate these findings. It is better to tell him in simple language what is wrong, instead of supplying him with "medical facts" which he can then cherish and, at the same time, misconstrue.

A chauffeur once consulted me for pains in his fingers, wrists and knees. Some well-meaning friend had told him that he had "arthritis." That just about finished him. He saw himself in a home for incurables, a hopeless, dependent invalid in a wheelchair. Well, he did not have arthritis and his quick recovery was due as much to my reassurance as to anything I prescribed for him.

Some patients disclaim any fear or worry, perhaps protesting too much. Others arrive at our offices with their chief complaints miraculously and suddenly gone. The illness need not, to be sure, give rise to any conscious anxiety in the patient, but this does not necessarily mean that no anxiety exists. Often the presence of anxiety betrays itself by the attitude toward the physician, who may quite unaccountably become the object of distrust and fear —fear that he may inflict pain, or perhaps tell us something we do not want to hear. We therefore begin to "blame" the doctor. For what? Ostensibly for being an alarmist, for being negligent, for coming too often, for not coming often enough, for telling us bad news about ourselves, for withholding bad news and, of course, for charging too much. Such attitudes on the part of patients and their relatives are familiar enough to all practicing physicians. They are not the result of mere cussedness, nor are they found only in those whom we label "neurotics"; they represent various common attempts to fend off anxiety. Like the Greeks, we want to kill the messenger who brings the bad tidings from Marathon. It is such attitudes that obstruct the early seeking of medical advice and hence the prevention of illness.

In my student days, when I was "doing obstetrics" in South

Boston, I dashed up the steps of a tenement and arrived just in time to hear the familiar inspiratory wail of a newborn infant. In the crude language of medical students, "She was a multip and I got a placenta," meaning that the mother, having had previous babies, had brought this one into the world in such a hurry that it arrived on the scene before I did. She looked at me indulgently and said: "I always like to have my babies before the doctor comes 'cause then you have none of them instruments." Such an attitude is not confined to obstetrical patients.

There are those who want to be brave; they carry on in spite of pain and discomfort; they do not like to make a fuss. It is not my intention to imply that a physician must be consulted for every minor ailment, but there are many complaints, as, for example, headache, fatigue and loss of weight, that indicate the need for a thorough examination.

Men are, by and large, much more careful of their cars than they are of themselves. At the first knock of the engine they will stop at a service station, or if the car is slow on the pickup or has lost power on an upgrade. Yet they themselves will puff and rattle along for months. They will tinker with their own bodies, depending for repairs on an odd assortment of advice and patent medicines. Of course, when our automobiles are out of order we have to have them repaired. Don't we use them to get to the station in the morning and to take the children to school? Besides, if we go to Frank's garage we can be pretty sure that he will find the trouble. He has a big supply of spare parts and he is an honest and reliable fellow. He said it would cost "somewhere in the neighborhood of twelve dollars," and we can depend on him not to stick us. Frank has one enormous advantage over us doctors. He can replace worn-out parts with new ones. The best we can do is to help the human machine to run as smoothly as it can until the last mile is ticked off. Of one thing you may be sure, however, the longer you wait the less we can do. The truth of this statement is especially obvious in mental and nervous disorders, in tuberculosis, in cancer, in the various heart afflictions, in diabetes and syphilis.

A man in moderate circumstances would not think it exorbitant to spend fifty or a hundred dollars a year on the upkeep of his car or even to add twice that sum for turn-in value on his old car. But if he has doctors' bills of these amounts he is sure to be pretty unhappy. Why are we so cheerfully willing to take care of our cars but not of ourselves, to pay out good money for their upkeep but to be niggardly and resentful about medical expenses?

To this question the conventional reply is that medical costs cannot be planned for. There is no room on the family budget for anything so incalculable as doctors' bills. Sickness is like a burst water main. It comes suddenly, an unheralded, unwelcome and unexpected act of God with which we are not prepared to cope. That is the usual argument.

I suspect, however, that our attitude toward the cost of medical care and toward periodic health examinations is greatly influenced by the irrationality in which this whole subject is shrouded. Actually, we are scared to think about being sick. We prefer to live our lives in the illusion of immortality. Time enough for moth and corruption after seventy-five! Who wants to go to the doctor just to be told that there's nothing wrong? Most normal, healthy adults do not take kindly to the thought of periodic physical examinations. Why is this? If they are vigorous, energetic people, hitting on all four cylinders, they do not want to be bothered. If they are past their peak they may choose to let sleeping dogs lie. It would only worry them to learn that their blood pressure was a little too high or that they had a trace of albumin in their urine. And yet there can be little doubt that regular yearly examinations would be of great advantage for the prevention of illness.

Dentists have succeeded better. Their "educated" patients come to them once or twice a year for prophylaxis, no longer waiting to be driven by toothache or gumboils. No one enjoys going to his dentist; we go in spite of pain and expense. After all, teeth are only teeth and whatever is wrong with them can involve no threat to our very being. No dentist can pronounce a death sentence.

In prenatal care and in the care of our children, too, we behave in a somewhat more rational manner. Here most intelligent people readily accept preventive procedures. It is customary for pregnant women to be examined at regular intervals until their babies are born. In the first few months of life the infant is seen every so often by a pediatrician and later in childhood periodic visits once or twice a year are customary among the so-called educated classes. Outlay of money for such professional services does not seem too great a burden. It is looked upon as a kind of insurance. When the responsibility is for someone else we do what we can to take precautions, but where we ourselves are concerned we need to overcome so much apprehension that we have a tendency to put off as long as possible the disagreeable ordeal of an examination which might disclose the awful truth.

It is obviously part of the doctor's job to help remove this massive anxiety which not only interferes with seeking early medical advice but also attributes false motives to the doctors and projects undeserved blame upon them, accentuating and distorting the matter of expense and putting obstacles in the way of periodic health examinations. Perhaps the first essential is for doctors themselves to understand the far-reaching consequences of this state of mind and to learn to recognize it in their individual patients—and deal with it. In addition the various medical associations and the life-insurance companies should put on a vigorous educational campaign urging periodic examinations. They should match radio plug with radio plug and for every car card peddling "Slim" for obesity and "Vim" for debility and "Him" for charm they should drive home the need for the ounce that prevents. In time such periodic examinations would become routine for the adult population, a good deal of the neurotic fear of them would disappear, and the bugaboo of expense would take its proper place.

There are probably certain additional psychological barriers against taking reasonable health precautions which might be lumped under the heading of indifference and inertia. I am told by an acquaintance of mine who practices medicine in the Texas cattle country that ranchers are quick to take advantage of modern veterinary science in having their herds tested for tuberculosis and protected against the ravages of such infections as Bang's disease and blackleg. But it would not occur to them to have their children examined or inoculated against smallpox, diphtheria or tetanus. Man has always been more concerned in safeguarding and preserving his property than his life.

As an example of the value of complete physical examinations the fact could be cited that out of approximately eighteen hundred apparently healthy women examined in two New York dispensaries one hundred and thirty-seven were discovered to have cancer—the majority in an early and curable stage. Without the health examinations the presence of malignant disease would probably not have been discovered until too late.

Such early detection of cancer rests not only upon periodic health examinations but requires, also, thoroughly trained physicians with the most modern facilities for early diagnosis at their disposal. What is true of cancer is true of many other serious diseases, and it is also true that the hospital provides the best setting for expert investigation.

Yet if there is anxiety associated with consulting a physician, how much more is there in going to a hospital? Every doctor who rode the ambulance in his youth recalls the beating of breasts and tearing of hair that accompanied the stretcher bearers' dreary trek down the tenement stairs.

After the last war I spent six months in eastern Macedonia helping to combat an epidemic of typhus fever among the natives. The Greeks who had been taken to Bulgaria during hostilities were repatriated in shiploads and housed in tobacco warehouses in the seaport of Kavalla. Typhus fever broke out on the ships and spread rapidly. In order to keep down the epidemic in Kavalla these unfortunates were quickly dispatched to their native towns and villages—carrying their lice with them. They were thoroughly frightened, and justly so, and resorted to various kinds of magic in order to avert the evil. Instead of submitting to delousing operations they chose the alternative of holding religious processions, led by a black-robed, black-bearded priest wearing a tall, black stovepipe hat and bearing the crucifix on high. And they hid their sick in cellars and attics and outhouses, often under bundles of rags from which we had to dig them out—anything rather than go to the typhus hospitals where they of course received much better care at the hands of the Greek medical officers and Red Cross nurses than they did at home. But they saw coffins carried out of the hospitals and felt sure that being sent there was equivalent to a death warrant. Perhaps one could have expected nothing else of these ignorant peasants who tilled their tobacco fields with wooden plowshares and drove solid-wheeled oxcarts. One often encounters a strikingly similar attitude in twentieth century New York. This is a great pity, because with all their defects and inefficiencies modern hospitals are the centers of medical knowledge and skill and the natural place for the great mass of people to turn to for help.

Isn't this the place to reflect upon a justifiable complaint of many hospital patients? I can't recall anyone of them ever claiming that the food was "delicious." In point of straight fact it is usually anything but. Why, with all the modern streamlined efficiency, need this most fundamental appetite and means to good health and pleasure be given such unimaginative attention? Just because invalid food should be simple, must it also be flat? Hospital superintendents and dieticians have, to be sure, done much to improve the quality of food and its proper balance, but no one will deny that more could be done to make the hospital meal a matter not only of good medicine but also of anticipatory and actual pleasure. While the doctors go home to a well-ordered dinner they often leave their patients to be comforted with custards, clabber, a lonely prune, or a slippery canned peach!

CHAPTER XVI

Office Practice, Hospitals and Outpatient Departments

IN THE preceding chapter I said that a good deal of the resistance against seeking medical advice and taking reasonable health precautions is based on what might justly be called neurotic anxiety. There are, however, some very real causes for misgivings on the part of the sick.

Take, for example, the case of Mr. Jones, the assistant sales manager of the Manhattan Hook and Eye Company. He lives in the suburbs with his wife and his boy and girl. Junior is in his last year at high school and Mr. and Mrs. Jones hope to send him to college. Sister is still in grammar school and is having her teeth straightened and taking piano lessons. Mrs. Jones had to have an operation last year. That was quite a blow to the family exchequer. But Jones is a steady, reliable man. He buys a bond every month, keeps up his life-insurance payments and is gradually amortizing the first mortgage on his house. He does not drink too much and has no vices except for an occasional evening of poker with the boys. On Saturdays he often goes to a ball game with the wife and kids. On rare occasions he and Mrs. Jones take in a show in town; that is, if they can hire a "sitter-in." He reads the *Saturday Evening Post*, *Reader's Digest* and *Time* and manages to keep up pretty well with what is going on in the world. He is too old to be in the war and his son is too young; so he considers himself pretty lucky. But he is doing his duty in his community. He has been active in civilian defense work and his wife is a nurse's aide—work she manages to do in spite of the shortage of help.

Recently he had to give up coffee. Just as he settles down to read his morning paper on the 8:05 he gets the most horrible heartburn. So he surreptitiously slips a few soda mints into his mouth. Last week when he made a tour of his territory in New England that dish of baked beans he ate in the restaurant at the South Station in Boston nearly killed him. He had something like this once before. It was about five years ago, just after he had been made assistant sales manager and had bought his house on the strength of his raise. Five thousand dollars looked pretty good to him then, but what with the increased cost of living and taxes there isn't much left at the end of the month. Still he has never been one to worry about money. There are more important things in the world than money. As long as the wife and kids are well and happy, he should worry! It's wonderful to see Junior developing the way he is. He won the prize for the best airplane model in the town hobby show. The kid is just crazy to fly. "I hope to God the war is over before he gets into the bloody mess. Damn it, there goes that pain again. I guess I'll run up to see Dr. Smith at lunchtime. He's said to be very clever, but he's awfully busy. I hope he'll be able to see me today."

Dr. Smith is a sober man graying toward fifty. He is about the same age as Jones. He has his worries too, but he has a good poker face. Smith takes a careful history. He was taught at medical school that the most important thing in diagnosing gastrointestinal complaints is taking a careful history. Smith's education did not stop at medical school. He attends meetings, reads medical journals and has even written a few papers. He has never specialized in stomach ailments and Jones wonders whether he shouldn't have gone directly to a big stomach man. In the meanwhile Smith is cogitating to himself: "It certainly sounds like a peptic ulcer, but it might be a gall bladder or just a gastric neurosis with hyperacidity. It's hard to tell. At Jones's time of life one always has to consider the possibility of a cancer, though it probably isn't one."

Jones isn't worried particularly—just fed up with the pain and he knows he can't afford to be sick. But Dr. Smith is a bit worried—in a professional way, of course. The man looks sick. His face is somewhat drawn and pale. Dr. Smith is a careful and kind clinician. He is self-possessed and assured and immediately inspires confidence in his patient. The last thing he wants to do is to frighten Jones and yet he knows that it's nothing to make light of. After a long series of questions lasting nearly half an hour he says something like this: "Mr. Jones, I'm not perfectly sure what you've got and I can't be until I've examined you further. Your story sounds more like a stomach ulcer than anything else. I want you to go on a diet and stick to it religiously for a week. That, together with some medicine I shall prescribe for you, which you are to take both before and after meals, should rid you of your indigestion and stop the pains. I should like you to come back to see me in four or five days. Remember, absolutely no departure from the diet and take your medicine regularly."

The doctor gives him an appointment for an examination and then shows him out. There is no mention of money and Jones isn't sure whether to pull out his wallet or not. Smith shakes hands with his patient and says a few reassuring words. There are several people waiting to see him. He is behind his schedule. He has to be at the Academy of Medicine at five o'clock for a committee meeting. He turns his mind to his next patient's problem. At least one gets the feeling in talking to Dr. Smith that he is attentive and wholly concerned with your troubles. So thinks Jones as he walks out of the doctor's office. But he is no longer Jones. Something new has been added. He is now John Jones plus an ulcer. He goes back to work and he is vaguely troubled. He hasn't any real pain but he catches an earlier train than usual. He takes a taxi home and surprises his wife. As soon as she looks at him she says: "Is anything wrong, darling?" He had intended not to tell her. But there's no use, he never could keep anything from her. He tells her about his visit to Dr. Smith and makes her promise not to say anything. Jones decides to take a nap before dinner. As soon as he is safely out of earshot Mrs. Jones goes to the telephone and calls up her sister: "John went to the doctor's this afternoon and he says he has stomach ulcers. [The public always prefers the plural.] Don't breathe it to a soul. Yes, he's going again on Tuesday for a thorough examination. Yes, I'll let you know what he says."

Dr. Smith leaves his office at five minutes to five. He steps into his car and as he drives toward the Academy his mind reflects on the afternoon's work. "That fellow Jones; I didn't like the way he looked. He's a decent sort—uncomplaining too. He seemed tense and worried. I doubt if he even knows that he's worried. I wonder whether there's anything in all this psychosomatic stuff. Maybe, but the first thing is a careful examination. I guess Dr. Brown will do a G.I. series on him for twenty-five dollars, or I could send him to the hospital for a semiprivate X-ray. He certainly can't afford the private-patient fee. It'll come to about the same in the end and most patients prefer going to private doctors. Brown is a damn decent fellow. He always asks me what to charge the patients I send him. He just did a public-school teacher for nothing. But then she's the sole support of her invalid mother. I charged her a minimum just for her self-respect."

Tuesday comes and Jones arrives fifteen minutes early. The doctor greets him and is a little disappointed to hear that his patient has had several bouts of pain in spite of following all directions. He takes him into the examining room and has him strip. Dr. Smith is businesslike and thorough. He looks a bit austere in his white coat and he examines his patient in a curiously objective way, dictating the while to his office nurse who takes it all down in shorthand. Jones is miffed to hear himself described as "well developed and poorly nourished." At least it's something to be well developed. He knows that he has lost about ten pounds in the last six months. His *sclerae* (which he learns later are the whites of his eyes) are not definitely *icteric* (the fancy word for jaundiced) but they are "muddy." (Here's mud in your eye!) Dr. Smith spends quite a lot of time groping around above the left collarbone. He seems to be looking for something he has lost. Finally he says to his nurse: "There is no *sentinel gland.*" ("Watchman, what of the night? What the heck is a sentinel gland?") When he comes to the abdomen, the doctor has a literary field day. He describes it as *scaphoid* or something like that and there is no *panniculus* of fat. That's lucky. Jones never did admire spare tires around the middle. There is no tenderness. (How does he know that?) Dr. Smith watches his patient's face intently while he presses gently but firmly on the pit of his stomach. Ah, yes, there is a tender area which makes him wince. So the good doctor presses again just to make sure. For a while Dr. Smith seems to go into a kind of trance. He shuts his eyes and runs the flat of his closed fingers again and again over the upper abdomen. Then he says dryly: "There are no masses or organs felt." (Jones, of course, doesn't know for sure whether that's good or bad.) The matter-of-fact physician pursues his relentless way. "The first and second fingers of the right hand are stained with tobacco. The knee jerks are equal and hyperactive." ("Well, at least I'm not crazy yet.") Then he is told to get dressed. The doctor washes his hands, takes off his white coat and returns to his consulting room to wait for his patient.

"Well," says the doctor, "the examination is essentially negative. You are a bit underweight and your hemoglobin and blood count are a little low. And I noticed in examining your prostate gland that it was rather large and hard, which could explain what you told me about having to get up to go to the bathroom two or three times at night. We must make some further investigations. First of all I want you to have an X-ray of your stomach and I'll try to see that it doesn't cost you too much." This is the first time money has been mentioned—though Jones has naturally had it pretty much on his mind. Jones says okay. If it must be, it must be. Then follows a brief telephone conversation with Dr. Brown, which begins with some mutual kidding. An appointment is arranged and the patient is instructed to report for X-ray examination three days later in the morning, without breakfast. Dr. Smith wants him to have an electrocardiogram as well and also to have his prostate examined by a genitourinary surgeon. It seems strange to him when his trouble is in his stomach, but the doctor knows best. Smith thereupon calls up another friend and there is a little more mutual kidding and another appointment is made. The doctor promises Jones that the electrocardiogram will not take long and assures him that it should not cost more than fifteen or twenty dollars at the most. He is to come back after the X-rays are completed. So Jones and his ulcer leave the office again—perhaps a little more troubled but feeling that he is in good hands.

Another visit. Dr. Smith is always his same calm and steady self. "Well, sir, your heart is okay. The electrocardiogram is perfectly normal. I wish mine were as good. But the X-ray pictures show a definite ulcer and also a defect in the filling of the stomach. So I guess we'll have to have your stomach washed out and, while we're at it, I think we'll have a squint inside with a gastroscope." "What's that?" asks Jones. "Oh, it's a new device by which they can actually look into your stomach. No, I can't do it myself but I'll send you to a colleague of mine who is extremely skillful. The whole thing won't cost you more than twenty-five dollars, including analysis of the stomach contents." ("Bang goes saxpence," says Jones to himself. "What the hell, I'll just have to sell a bond.") "By the way, doctor, what is your fee?"

Now Smith is a kind man and he's not out for money, but he has a wife and children of his own to support and insurance and taxes and office expenses. It costs him close on to five thousand dollars a year for the privilege of practicing. So he says: "I'll try to make it reasonable for you. I'll charge you ten dollars for the first visit and ten dollars for the physical examination and five dollars for subsequent visits. I'll have to charge you extra for laboratory tests." Jones says: "That's very good of you, doctor, I appreciate it"—and then to himself: "Twenty-five and twenty-five and twenty and twenty-five."

And another visit. Jones is definitely better, and the pain is less frequent than it was. Dr. Smith: "I hate to put you through more tests but, as I told you, I think you should have your prostate checked up on. You know we're getting to the age when some men begin to have trouble. Naturally that hasn't anything to do with your stomach, but while we're at it we might as well shoot the works." So Dr. Smith reaches for the telephone. He calls his friend Black: "She had a what?—a dermoid cyst with hair and teeth in it? Well, I'll be damned! By the way, Bill, will you see a patient for me? I'll call you later and talk to you about him. You have no time till next week? Just a minute. [To Jones]: He says he can't see you till next week." The ulcer and Jones leave the office. Only his respect for Dr. Smith and his confidence in him keep him from muttering: "What the hell is this anyway, a run-around?"

If any doctor should happen to read these pages he will have guessed what Dr. Smith has in mind and why he is being so careful. He is not perfectly certain that his patient hasn't a cancer of the stomach and he cannot take any chances. He has to make assurance doubly sure. It may be a matter of life and death for Jones, and Jones has a lot to live for. Naturally he's not going to make his patient's days and nights miserable by betraying his own misgivings, and he cautions his surgical friend not even to mention the possibility of an operation on the prostate. He doesn't want to add to Jones's troubles.

Dr. Black, the surgeon, is chunky and vigorous. He is snappier than Smith and moves more quickly and surely. He hasn't the sad and contemplative look of a man who frequently beholds the spectacle of human suffering without being able to do much about it. His inquiries are more pointed and his examination is pretty much limited to the area in question. Dr. Black bows the patient out. He says very little except that he will report directly to Dr. Smith.

Another visit to Dr. Smith. The gnawing sensation which Jones complained of in his stomach is less troublesome. But he is worried, chiefly because his wife keeps asking him what the doctor says and he doesn't know just what to tell her. Dr. Smith looks a bit haggard and tired today. He says to Jones: "My friend Black agrees with me that there is nothing really wrong with your prostate." ("I never thought there was," says Jones to himself.) The doctor then makes one or two changes in the diet and allows his patient to go after a short and, on the whole, reassuring call.

Another visit. Jones feels more at ease with his doctor, who greets him warmly. The two men have come to like each other. The doctor says: "Everything's okay. The gastroscopic examination showed nothing unexpected, nor did the stomach contents. I guess I was right in the first place. You've got a simple peptic ulcer. If you keep on as you have and take it a little easier it ought to be healed up in a few months. Perhaps in six months or so we'll have another X-ray, just to make sure everything's all right." "Okay, Doc," says the assistant sales manager of the Manhattan Hook and Eye Company, "anything but that damned sword swallowing. Once was enough."

Jones recovers. In six months there is no longer any X-ray evidence of an ulcer. He has put on weight and his color is better. His stomach rarely kicks up, only when there are too many orders to fill or when the bottom drops out of the Hook and Eye market. He has made a friend of Smith who allows him to pay off his debt in monthly installments. The whole thing came to about two hundred dollars, which is fair enough, even though it is too little to be tax deductible.

At the beginning of this chapter I spoke of some very real causes for misgivings on the part of the sick. Now, why should our friend Jones have cause for misgivings over the treatment he received? He got the best that medical science and skill have to offer and certainly the cost was not too staggering. But he was in luck. By the merest chance he fell into the hands of a well-trained, conscientious and considerate doctor. In fact, he was initiated into a kind of medical club: Dr. Smith and his friend Brown, the X-ray man, and Black, the urologist and the others—all decent, fine fellows with hospital connections, all working together, doing favors for each other and adjusting their fees to meet his modest income. Most of the "better men" in medicine are willing to do that. But, obviously, if Smith treated too many Joneses at a reduced fee, his own income would soon fall off. If he cut down his overhead, dispensed with his office nurse and moved to a less desirable part of town, he would soon lose his well-to-do clientele. And if he saw more patients for less money he could no longer conduct the exemplary type of practice that he does. Supposing Jones had consulted one of those high-priced specialists with a flat fee for everybody—exceptions though they may be—one who never charges less than twenty-five dollars. Or supposing Jones had gone to some obscure physician without hospital connections, without a circle of trusted colleagues to call upon for help. It might have cost him only two dollars a visit. But could he have had the painstaking physical examination, the X-rays and laboratory studies and the various consultations? Most certainly not. Were they really necessary? Couldn't he have been cured without all that stuff? Perhaps so. I believe, however, and I suspect that most medicos will agree with me, that our job is more than just to perpetrate "cures." We have to know what we are curing. We have to prevent recurrences and complications—in Jones's case hemorrhage and perforation; and, of course, if we want to save lives, we have to detect anything like a cancer as early as possible. This is the least that should be expected of sound medical practice. Perhaps I have said enough to indicate why Jones should scratch his head in wonder at the complexity of what had originally seemed to him so simple—a pain in the stomach.

Now let us look at the other side. For some months now Jones has not been able to read the fine type in the telephone book; his arms do not seem to be quite long enough. His medical expenses have been high and he wants to save money, so he presents himself at the eye clinic of one of our best hospitals—one with a liberal policy about accepting patients of Jones's income level. After all, he is an enlightened man. He knows that a modern hospital bears little resemblance to the place of woe and torment of the last century. So there he is awaiting his turn to be interviewed by the admitting nurse. After the interview, Jones proceeds to the cashier and waits in line to pay his admission fee. Next he must find his way up to the typist in the middle of the corridor on the floor above. He sits on another bench waiting his turn with the typist. To her he dictates a lot of information which she types onto the face sheet of his medical record about the date of his birth, his nationality, marital status, father's birthplace, mother's maiden name and so on. He then proceeds to the eye clinic, registers at the desk and has a seat on the bench until his name is called, whereupon a technician takes all new eye patients into the Sorting Room to perform a preliminary vision test and take a brief history of each patient's eye complaint. He waits again on a bench in the Sorting Room until there are enough new patients (ten or fifteen) to make it worthwhile for the doctor to come over. The doctor examines Jones very briefly to determine to which section of the eye clinic he is to be sent. This examination is too hurried to give him the feeling of really having been seen by a doctor. Jones is instructed to go back to the cashier, pay a dollar for the refraction, and then report to the Vision Room, where he again warms a bench for a while. He is called to the desk to be told by the Vision Room secretary that refractions are not done the same day that they are ordered and that no appointments are available for at least a week. The secretary gives him an appointment and his prescription for drops and written instructions about how to use them. Jones takes his prescription downstairs to the apothecary where he pays for the medicine and waits quite a long time before the drops are ready. During the course of the morning our friend has sat waiting on six separate benches and has seen a doctor for a little less than six minutes. If he has a headache by the time he goes out to lunch I suspect it won't be due solely to his eye trouble.

This schedule is an actual one from the outpatient department of one of our best "voluntary" teaching hospitals, distinguished for its fine humanitarian tradition, with none of the cattle-pen atmosphere of some of our overcrowded, understaffed city dispensaries. It was furnished me by an unusually intelligent and observing young woman. The routine described is manifestly uneconomical and not designed to achieve the desired results. It lacks imagination. No industrial engineer would think of testing radio tubes or automobile tires in such a wasteful manner. Viewed only from the standpoint of efficiency it surely is not the best way of testing eyes, even if we leave out of consideration common human needs. But common human needs cannot be left out if we want to achieve good results. The excuse is, of course, that there is no money available. Funds are insufficient. There is also the convention that beggars mustn't be choosers and that the poor should be satisfied with what we give them. Their small clinic fee does not begin to pay for the overhead of running the department, and the busy doctors contribute their services without recompense.

In the best of our outpatient departments, when the case load per doctor is not too great, patients can get excellent medical care. There are some in which they are seen by appointment only. New ones are given as much as forty-five minutes for the first examination and return cases are allowed at least fifteen minutes. Sometimes the same doctor follows a group of patients for many years, an arrangement making for continuity of treatment and for confidence in the clinic.

At the other extreme is the herding and crowding process.

With one eye on the clock the overworked doctor is impatient of neurotic complaints, constituting, as it is certain they do, the bulk of the troubles he has to deal with. Although physical examination may be adequate enough, history taking, the most important part in many diagnoses, is skimped and routinized. Return patients are quickly disposed of with a renewal of their old prescriptions and have to get satisfaction from a fresh bottle of "No. 253," which probably contains a small amount of potassium iodide or chloral or bromides or cascara. They are comforted by the magic fluid. It makes them feel better. But they may have a sense of having been cheated, and justly so—cheated of the most important item a doctor has to dispense: his time, his care and his interest. Good medicine cannot be practiced in a hurry, or impersonally.

Naturally it costs more to run a clinic on a sound time schedule with a reasonable case load, but such a system is greatly to be desired for all clinics if the public is to reap the benefits of modern medicine.

For people of low incomes the outpatient clinic has many advantages over a private physician. At a reasonable fee they can receive the benefit not only of a general examination and special laboratory tests and X-rays but also advice and treatment at the hands of specialists, some of them leaders in their fields. As I pointed out in the first chapter of this book, often it is no longer possible for one medical man to take all the necessary technical steps for arriving at a satisfactory diagnosis. And some complicated forms of treatment can be administered only by specialists who possess the required training and equipment. In a sense all good medical practice has become co-operative. A doctor who manages his own office nevertheless works in collaboration with others, if he is conscientious. He will be in constant touch with surgeons, neurologists, "nose and throat men," and from time to time he will need various kinds of technical assistance. But consultations in private practice are costly and time consuming and involve the patient in a good deal of running around.

What we need are widely scattered diagnostic centers where the best that medical science has to offer is available to everyone. Today these are sadly lacking in many communities. Furthermore the attendant medical staffs and technicians should be paid for their services. All aroma of sweet charity should be cleared from the air. These centers should be planned and administered with an eye to accuracy and efficiency of work and economy of time. The American genius for mass production and assembly-line technology should be brought to bear on this important problem. Any doctor should be able to refer his patients to such a center to get help with his diagnostic and therapeutic problems.

Some of my medical confreres are fond of boasting that we in the United States have the lowest sickness rate of any country in the world. Even if this boast could be substantiated by statistical data it does not justify a smug satisfaction with the present state of medical practice, whose most important task is to prevent illness and to discover disease at its beginning. Nothing would facilitate this more than the establishment of diagnostic centers all over the land—for rich and middle class and poor. Whether they are to be supported by voluntary contributions, or by pooling the resources in a community and sharing risks, or by grants-in-aid from the state or from the federal government is, for the present, beside the point.

The essence of good medical care depends, in my opinion, upon a closer relationship between the patient and a doctor with a healing personality, one who cares about helping him and who has at his disposal all the technical facilities of twentieth-century medicine. Neither by itself is sufficient. Only a combination of the two will produce the desired results.

CHAPTER XVII

Socialized Medicine or Paying the Piper

NOT long ago I paid a visit to my dentist. He had me properly trussed up and gagged, with rubber dam, gurgling syphon and the rest. In the midst of his manipulations he stopped long enough to ask: "Doctor, do you believe in socialized medicine?" I thought: "You're pretty smart! You spring the question on me unprepared, gagged and garroted as I am, and then proceed to expound your views."

It is a question frequently posed these days, and as frequently answered without much regard to the meaning of the two words. At the risk of pedantry I should like to define them because then at least we shall know what we can agree or disagree about. The word *medicine* is an omnibus. It includes the whole elaborate structure of teaching and research. It includes hospital administration and the training of nurses. It includes the science of sanitation, the inspection of food, the supervision of drug manufacture and sales. It includes the public-health services, quarantining and control of contagious diseases, institutional care of the mentally ill and of the tuberculous. It includes maternal care and the prevention of infant mortality. It includes medical jurisprudence, the licensing of physicians and, finally, the practice of the healing arts. It is only the last of these that the layman usually thinks of in connection with medicine.

Now by the word *socialized* as it is applied to medicine, we mean, so it seems to me, some kind of governmental planning and control of these various functions. Again we must stop to define *governmental,* which may refer to municipal planning and control, to county, or to state, or to federal.

In this country at the present time much of medicine is already socialized. Towns and municipalities of any considerable size have their departments of health and sanitation to supervise water supply and sewage disposal, to collect and record statistics on the causes of death. They have their laboratories devoted to the study and prevention of infections and contagions. City hospitals and dispensaries are operated at the taxpayers' expense. In New York City the combined budgets of the departments of health, hospitals and sanitation for the year 1944–45 were in excess of seventy-three million dollars. In many counties there are sanitaria for the treatment of the tuberculous, and there is no state in the Union that has not made some provision—inadequate though it often is—for the care of the mentally sick, the feeble-minded and the criminally insane. At least three-quarters of the total number of hospital beds in the United States are paid for out of public funds.

The United States Public Health Service, even during times of peace, operates on a budget of some fifty million dollars and concerns itself with many public-health problems that are of an interstate nature, the quarantining of vessels and the inspection of immigrants, for example. It provides funds and lends personnel to the various states for important public-health projects such as venereal disease control. Medical care of the merchant marine and coast guard is one of its many functions, as well as the operation of several large hospitals. One of these is St. Elizabeth's in Washington, D. C., a sixty-eight-hundred-bed institution devoted to the care of mental illness, and there are others for the treatment of narcotic addicts. It is forever vigilant against the importation of such diseases as Asiatic cholera, bubonic plague, yellow fever, typhus and trachoma. It conducts a ceaseless battle with the carriers of certain diseases: with the hookworm, with the malarial mosquito, with rats and other rodents that may harbor fleas that can convey bubonic plague and with ticks that may be infected with rickettsia, the organism that transmits Rocky Mountain spotted fever. These parasites are no respecters of state boundaries. Only a federal authority can deal with them effectively.

Socialized medicine in this country is therefore nothing new. It is an accomplished fact. Medicine has been socialized only, however, in those departments having to do with diseases or illnesses that are menacing to society—dangerous contagions or infections, serious psychiatric disorders, for example. In addition, in local communities, the care of the poor—sometimes called the medically indigent—has become the concern and charge of those communities.

The issue at stake is, shall medicine be *further* socialized? Shall government planning and control, at the local, state or federal levels, be allowed to invade our privately endowed medical schools and hospitals, our research institutions, and especially—by a system of compulsory insurance—the private practice of medicine? This is the embattled front in organized medical societies. This is where blood begins to boil, where friendships break, where high explosives are dropped. It is for you to decide what kind of medical care you want and how you are going to pay for it. Only, do not be deceived into believing that a system of easy payments will solve the problem of good medical care or that it can emerge out of a political football scrimmage. All I can do is to give you my opinion as to what constitutes *good medical care.* I am not an economist or a sociologist or a political reformer. I am a doctor. As such it is my interest and purpose to see to it that the patients whom I treat are well treated, that they do not become financially ruined in the process and that I myself can earn a decent living from my work. This is the issue, at least as it concerns private practice, reduced to its simplest elements.

But we are not quite ready yet to discuss private practice. First I should like to analyze the source of the heat and fury, to blow away the smoke and see where the fire is. Dr. So-and-so No. One, an important man both in his profession and in so-called organized medicine, makes a speech at a dinner for influential (i.e., wealthy) laymen. He says: "No country which has permitted the federal subsidy of medicine has thereafter produced scientific work of any consequence." Whereupon Dr. So-and-so No. Two—a literal-minded fellow—writes to his colleague and says: "How come, Doctor? How about Pavlov's work which went on all through the darkest days of terror in the Russian Revolution? The government gave him food for his dogs when children were starving."

"Well, of course, if you want Bolshevism over here, that's something else. If you think it's more important to feed dogs than children, then I know what kind of man I'm talking to."

"Was Pavlov's work important or was it not? How about the researches of the Kaiser Wilhelm Gesellschaft, supported by the Kultusministerium in Germany? How about the discovery of such drugs as avertin and the sulfa derivatives?"

"So you are arguing for totalitarianism over here, are you? Well, I never thought you were that sort. You know what the Krankenkasse did to the practice of medicine in Germany. Bismarck started all the trouble. It was his way of anesthetizing the lower classes. We don't want any such methods in a democracy. They're not consistent with our way of life."

"How about Sir H. H. Dale's studies in pharmacology supported by the Medical Research Council of Great Britain — and all the important work done in England on influenza?"

"You know as well as I do that the British Medical Society is highly dissatisfied with the panel system. Why, an English country doctor can no longer call his soul his own. He has to treat patients he doesn't want to treat and he is nearly swamped with paper work. No sirree, sir, not for me; once you let 'em get their foot in the door, I tell you, man, you're licked. Why, I'll simply shut up shop. I'd rather raise potatoes on my farm in Maine."

And so it goes. This is the rub—the rub that lights the sparks, that kindles the fire, that generates the heat, that fills your eyes with smoke. There is no meeting of minds. There are no sharply defined issues. We charge windmills, wrestle with ghosts and run our bayonets through straw men.

I often think it comical, as did red-coated Private Willis while pacing up and down before his sentry box: "How nature always does contrive that ev'ry boy and ev'ry gal that's born into the world alive is either a little Liberal or else a little Conservative! Fal, lal—la! Fal, lal—la!"

How is there ever to be a meeting of minds, especially when the embattled cohorts get behind their respective prejudices and hurl epithets at each other? It was Robert Frost, I believe, who said: "I never dared be a radical in my youth for fear I should be a conservative in my old age."

The issues here are no different from those confronting the rest of society: those of minorities, pressure groups, the democratic process and the good old steam roller. Only doctors, as a class, are not very adept at the great game of politics.

As I have intimated, all the familiar slogans and shibboleths come to the fore: "States' rights *vs.* centralization; supply and demand; distribution of commodities." "Starving in the midst of plenty." "Government interference; bureaucracy; getting something for nothing." "What will they expect next—to have the government pay for our drinks?" "Free enterprise; rugged individualism; normalcy." "Lowering of standards." "Can a handful of social reformers tell us how to manage a case of encephalitis lethargica?" "Work on a salary? I should say not!" "Do you know what the average income is in the United States? Do you know that one catastrophic illness can ruin a family?" "I don't want any government agent telling me what to charge my patients or how to treat them, either." "They make me sick—they tell us to take the initiative, to live up to our social responsibilities. Is there any other profession that works so hard, that gives so much for nothing? And then they accuse us of not being socially minded!"

"Horse and buggy doctors; horse and buggy minds. This is the twentieth-century man. Be air-minded. Why, there'll be airplane ambulances as big as the B–29's. They'll be flying the sick to strategically placed medical centers." "Assembly-belt, processing sausage machine." "It's the personal relationship that counts and the free choice of your own physician. They'll be picking your wife for you next."

Puff, puff. Let's blow away the smoke again. It is no new idea that the world we live in is rapidly changing. One hundred years ago four out of five gainfully employed persons were independent farmers, craftsmen or merchants. Today four out of five are wage earners or salaried employees, depending for their jobs on the labor market. This change alone has brought with it a good deal of insecurity. As a corrective measure for this insecurity we have introduced various insurance measures against unemployment, disability, old age and death, which aim to mitigate the hardships of uncertain employment and to prevent depressions. They are not the work of hair-brained social reformers and doctrinaire professors but the logical and inevitable accompaniments of an industrialized society. These reforms have probably come to stay no matter whether, in the political zodiac, the sun passes through the sign of the donkey or the elephant. Such reforms are not indigenous to our climate. In one country after another a point is reached when there is a tremendous demand for social protection: Germany, England, France, Switzerland, Holland, Scandinavia. And now here. It has come late. As long as the country was thinly populated, as long as there was open land, a large immigration —with gold rushes and the enormous potential wealth of an expanding economy—the need was not felt. Now there is little free land, no immigration. We have come to live in a highly industrialized society and with it has come social-security legislation.

The technological revolution has not only affected industry and our habits and manner of living; it has also wrought profound changes in the practice of medicine which has experienced its own technological revolution due to the growth and development of medical science. Some of these changes I have tried to outline in previous chapters. Among the many results from which we all benefit daily, there are also certain disadvantages. The cost of adequate medical care has mounted greatly in the last few decades. Medicine has more to give than people are able to receive; just as with food, about half the population of the world suffers from malnutrition—if not from actual famine—in the face of plenty. As yet our social organization has not kept pace with the requirements of science.

It has been estimated that the average cost for complete medical care lies somewhere between $25.30 and $66.97 per person per year. In 1930 the annual outlay for medical care (exclusive of dentistry and drugs) for all income groups averaged only $16.86 per person. Approximately $8.00 per person were spent by families earning under $1,200, as contrasted with $82 by families earning $10,000 or more.

Now in normal times roughly 50 per cent of all American families have incomes of less than $1,500 a year and about 80 per cent have incomes of less than $3,000. Average incomes per family for 1928 (before the crash) were given as $2,116; for 1939, $2,267.

According to the testimony of the American Medical Association all families making up to $3,000 a year need assistance in meeting the cost of serious illness. It has been estimated that one family in a hundred is crippled by the cost of illness. If we break down incomes into several groups the story is something like this: Families with incomes of $4,500 can usually manage to meet the cost of severe illness by drawing on savings or by borrowing—it is stated that 30 per cent of all personal loans are made to cover the cost of illness. Families whose incomes lie between $4,500 and $2,000 can pay usual costs but cannot meet emergency expenses. Those with incomes of $2,000 to $750 cannot meet ordinary costs, or are barely able to do so. Families existing on less than $750 must obviously be taken care of at the public expense.

Now, one need not be a mathematical genius or a certified public accountant to see at once that the average American family is out of luck as far as getting good medical care is concerned. They certainly will not spend a nickel for it that they don't have to. All our fine plans for periodic health examination, for early detection of disease, for corrective orthopedic work in childhood, for widespread mental hygiene, even for reasonable dental care will go aglimmering if the facts stated above are true. And they are true.

What of the converse of this picture? What of the income of physicians? One could almost predict it even if the facts were not available.

A study was made of the incomes of 3,810 general practitioners for the year 1928. Twenty-eight earned more than $30,000; the average net income, however, for the whole group was estimated to be $5,250—an average naturally raised by the few with large incomes. Half earned net incomes under $4,400 and a quarter under $3,000. Similar studies with similar findings were made in 1936 and 1941.

In other words most general practitioners themselves fall into the category of persons who cannot afford to pay for medical care. It is true that doctors do not customarily charge one another or their dependents. Let us remember, however, that the doctor's bill is by no means the largest item of medical expense. There are hospital bills to pay, operating-room, X-ray and laboratory fees, costs for nursing care, for drugs and appliances. All of these costs have had a tendency to rise with the cost of living. The doctor's fee, however, is expected not to go up. Instead the public exerts a steady pressure on him actually to reduce his fee, because it is the one element in the scale of expenses which is not fixed, which has remained elastic and is, therefore, susceptible to bargaining. Doctors are poor bargainers, and besides most of them do not like the role.

Given the facts I have presented, then, one might logically conclude that in normal times there are millions of persons who cannot afford to employ doctors and that there are thousands of doctors who cannot make a decent living. The war, of course, has "solved" the problem of unemployment among doctors as it has among industrial workers. One unthinking solution offered during peacetime is to reduce the number of doctors! Then the remaining ones would have more to do. But the number of doctors should be determined not by their capacity to earn a living but by the health needs of a community.

We had 151,000 practicing doctors in this country before Pearl Harbor (not including 7,500 interns) and our total population was nearly 132,000,000. That comes to about one doctor for every 880 people.

The ratio, naturally, varies greatly in different sections of the country. Actually as the average income per person decreases, the number of persons per physician increases. For New York State it is 1 to 487, for Mississippi 1 to 1,700. These are, of course, prewar figures. A ratio of one doctor to 800 persons is considered satisfactory under normal conditions. In the military it is about 1 to 150.

Good medical care depends, however, as I have repeatedly pointed out, upon modern diagnostic and therapeutic installations, as well as upon the presence of a suitable number of practitioners. Such installations are far from evenly divided among the states. There are many sections of the country where an X-ray apparatus, for example, cannot be found. In New York State there is one bed in a general hospital for every 263 individuals, in Mississippi one for every 667. Approximately 1,200 counties with a population in excess of 15,000,000 persons have no recognized hospital facilities.

What, then, of the state of the nation? The Selective Service

System has given us more than a random sampling of the nation's health. It might be assumed that the younger men of the country represent the pick of the crop. At least they do not suffer from the disabilities of middle life, from the so-called degenerative diseases to which I have alluded in an earlier chapter. And yet the facts revealed, and now made public before a United States senatorial subcommittee, are appalling. Over 4,100,000 draft registrants, aged eighteen through thirty-seven, have been rejected as unfit for military service, discarded from a pool of approximately 13,000,000 (June 1, 1944). This makes the rejection rate nearly one out of every three men examined. Of course, there were many selected in spite of physical defects, which were present in eight out of every ten registrants. A higher rejection rate occurred in rural than in urban areas, except in such states as, for example, Minnesota and Wisconsin where there are relatively high incomes and good medical facilities. Draft rejections were highest in the states of the southeast where the lowest incomes and poorest medical facilities coexist.

According to the testimony before this committee a large proportion (15 to 20 per cent) of defects disqualifying registrants for military services were remediable (one out every six of the total men examined had a remediable defect)—among them, venereal diseases, hernias and dental defects. Some of course cannot be corrected even by the best medical care. Our concern here is not with them, however, but with those that can be corrected.

Captain C. R. Wells, U.S.N.R., Chief Dental Officer of the Selective Service System, stated that 95 per cent of the American people are in need of dental care at all times and that only some 30 per cent of those in need of it get adequate care. This figure corresponds pretty well to the one given above on annual incomes for families in normal times: only 25 per cent having incomes above $3,000.

By using army dentists on three eight-hour shifts per day, a stupendous dental-rehabilitation program is being carried out, making use of as much as three and a half times the dental equipment normally used each year for the entire population.

The army has, moreover, inducted and treated nearly 140,000 men with venereal infections, previously classified as 4F.

According to the National Health Survey (1938) there were 23,500,000 persons in the United States suffering from chronic diseases or physical impairments; and the United States Public Health Service surveys showed that industrial workers lose on an average of ten to twelve days a year because of illness. It is claimed that more man-hours are sacrificed each year because of gonorrhea and syphilis, both preventable and curable diseases, than because of strikes. The annual loss to America's productive effort due to physical disability is said to be a billion man-days, representing an aggregate waste of some ten billion dollars.

In the face of these facts does it seem particularly cogent, after all, to keep complacently repeating that we enjoy the lowest rate of sickness and the finest health service of any country in the world? Such an assertion does not become true by mere reiteration. Our superiority is more hope than fact. Even the most ardent devotee of the status quo will be given pause by the evidence uncovered by the Selective Service System. Indeed, the need for improvement seems now to be pretty generally recognized by the public, by the more liberal elements in our profession and recently, even, by the die-hards among us. But there is still a good deal of difference of opinion as to what should be done.

Looking at the problem in broad terms, the trouble seems to be that although medicine has fine wares to sell, they cost too much, and that therefore vast numbers of persons cannot afford to buy them. The rich can buy them; the poor get them for nothing or almost nothing, but the office worker, farm hand, factory employee, schoolteacher, small shopkeeper, often get either inferior goods or go without. Some provision is necessary to insure medical care for the masses.

That the need is felt and recognized and that something is being done to meet it is evident from what has actually taken place during the last few decades. Just as modern industry has grown from individual craftsmen through guilds to labor unions and eventually to highly organized units for mass production, so medicine seems to be developing. The doctor with his little black bag was once the sole dispenser of the healing art, like the cobbler who sat patiently and even lovingly over his last. Certainly shoes would be too costly today if they were made in the old way, and there would not be nearly enough to go around. Though the individual doctor is still the essential unit in good medical care, there is a tendency for him to join with others not only for the purpose of pooling knowledge and mutual education but also in order that his services may reach more people.

After the last war, groups of private practitioners—especially in the west and midwest—organized "firms" in the manner of lawyers. This system has not yet spread widely. Too often the older and more experienced man in the group was a prima donna, on whose virtuosity the rest of the cast depended, and with his death the group sometimes disbanded. The same period saw the growth of some of our most successful privately owned clinics. These resulted from the labors of specially gifted and brilliant men whose services were of such value and in such demand that they had to be organized and institutionalized in order to dispense them efficiently. I refer to such units as the Crile Clinic in Cleveland, the Lahey Clinic in Boston, the Mayo Clinic in Rochester, Minnesota, and to others less generally known. The superior work of these men and their staffs has served as a model of excellence and efficiency. Their fees were put on a businesslike basis, proportionate to the patient's income.

Large university teaching hospitals developed—supported in the main by voluntary contributions—some of them housed in enormous plants representing millions of dollars of capital investment. These medical centers provide in many respects the most expert, skillful and humane care that we have as yet achieved and can serve as models for any future system of less expensive medical care. However, they have not yet addressed themselves successfully to the problem of reduced cost for the great middle class or to a constructive policy toward health preservation. They deal, in the main, with the sick only. They dispense charity. A ward patient pays one-third to one-half of what it costs to maintain him. The resulting deficit is in part made good by disproportionate charges on the well-to-do (just as in private practice) and in part by the munificence of rich men, and often out of the budgets of universities which today are beginning to assume responsibility for the application of learning to social needs. There are also public funds available for patients who cannot meet the minimum rates. Semiprivate accommodations are too limited in numbers and the costs are still much too high.

The inevitable result of all this has been to apply the principles of prepayment insurance to the costs of medical care. I should like to state right now that no system of easier and less painful payments, no act of Congress, will in itself insure good medical care, which must always depend upon good doctors and enough of them, and upon good hospitals and enough of them also. There are clearly two problems involved: the first has to do with what constitutes good medical care and the second with how to make it generally available. Now if doctors know anything, they ought to know something about the first problem; but neither by training nor by interest can they contribute much to the second. The paradox of the situation is that doctors are busying themselves with the actuarial minutiae, and sociologists, statisticians, politicians and government officials are busying themselves with details of medical care. Perhaps we will make steadier and more rapid progress when the experts begin to cooperate, each staying in his own field.

In the sixty years before 1910 American health insurance had hardly started. Certain plans in limited areas, especially in the mining, lumber and railroad industries, had come into being, but they were mostly in the nature of indemnities for loss of time and injury. There were also plans for sickness insurance underwritten by fraternal societies, by mutual-benefit associations of employees and by trade unions. By 1911 workmen's compensation laws were introduced in many of the industrial states. These laws held the employers liable for injuries through accidents suffered by workers on the job. After that a drive for compulsory health insurance was organized by the American Association for Labor Legislation, but by 1920 it had died. It was opposed by organized medicine, commercial insurance companies and other powerful business interests. Organized labor was itself at the time divided on the question of compulsory health-insurance legislation, while today it is wholeheartedly behind it, but the other forces are as opposed now as they were then.

With the failure to introduce compulsory insurance came the rise of voluntary, prepayment, group-health-insurance plans. The risks of writing insurance for individuals, who are often people aware of their need for benefits, are greatly reduced by underwriting groups. A substantial reduction of costs is achieved by the inclusion of enough healthy persons to support the sick ones. These plans have stimulated employers to participate in paying the premiums.

In 1929 nonprofit hospitalization insurance began in a single hospital in Dallas, Texas. It spread rapidly, was accepted by the American Hospital Association and adopted as a means of dealing with the desperate financial plight that the years of depression had brought to many of our voluntary hospitals. By 1943 there were seventy-seven such Blue Cross plans with over twelve million subscribers. Most of them insure against the cost of room and board in semiprivate accommodations for a limited number of days per year. Some comprise plans for care on wards at reduced rates and make allowances for the costs of X-rays and laboratory work and for the use of operating rooms and anesthetics. For such insurance the expenses are approximately ten dollars a year for a single person, eighteen dollars for two persons and twenty-four dollars for a family, if enrollment is on a group basis. These costs do not cover the services of physicians and surgeons.

There are (since 1930), however, many voluntary plans in operation for pooling and spreading risks and costs in the payment of doctors' bills. In thirteen states such plans exist with the approval or under the sponsorship of official medical societies. They have a total enrollment of over a million subscribers. Some three hundred voluntary prepayment insurance plans have been instituted. Coverage varies from plan to plan but is most frequently aimed at the most dramatic items of medical expense: surgical operations and obstetrical care. The cost per individual and family is approximately the same as for hospitalization: twenty-four dollars a year for a family including husband, wife and children under eighteen.

In normal times, or during depressions, with family incomes at the low levels described above, such costs would probably prohibit any widespread subscriptions. The great majority of the population is still totally uninsured and coverage does not as yet, in most cases, include ordinary medical expenses, health examinations, nursing care or dentistry. Such complete coverage would naturally raise the costs.

One plan for fairly complete medical care now in operation exists at the Ross-Loos Clinic in Los Angeles, California. This clinic has approximately twenty-seven thousand prepaid subscribers and an additional seventy-five thousand dependents. The subscribers pay thirty dollars a year and get in return complete doctors' services in office, home and hospital, including preventive and general care and all specialist services. Hospitalization up to ninety days in a ward is assured, with ambulance service, X-ray, laboratory tests, drugs and dressings. Special nursing and maternity care and dental care are not provided. The dependents are charged fees ranging from fifty cents for an office call to twenty-five dollars for a major operation. There is no income limitation among the subscribers but the majority are in the white-collar groups. One hundred full-time physicians comprise the staff and from among them the subscribers may choose their own doctors. The excellence of the medical service rendered by the Ross-Loos Clinic has been attested to by no less an authority than Dr. Henry E. Sigerist, of Johns Hopkins.

Another plan that has attracted a good deal of public attention is that of the Permanente Foundation for Henry J. Kaiser's shipbuilding employees. The coverage and costs are almost identical with the Ross-Loos plan but there is no provision for dependents. The Kaiser organization has built, on the proceeds of its subscriptions, large modern hospital buildings with all the latest medical equipment.

None of the plans thus far described represents a "socialization" of medicine in the sense that either local, state or federal government has had a hand in it. A second drive in this direction is now emergent. It has had its origin in the changing social philosophy of our times and more specifically in the Social Security Act of 1935, from which health insurance was the only major form of security to be omitted. In 1939 Senator Wagner proposed a bill amending the act to include health security, but it was not passed by Congress. Organized labor has insisted on further protection, and this has resulted in a new bill, known as S–1161, which is now pending. It is also known as the Wagner-Murray-Dingell Bill. It proposes to include practically the entire population, regardless of income, for all the major items of medical expense except dentistry, drugs and home nursing. Medical service is to be paid for by payroll deductions of 3 per cent and employer contributions of a like amount on wages or salaries up to three thousand dollars. The bill, though strongly supported by the A.F. of L. and the C.I.O., is opposed with bitterness by the American Medical Association, which holds that the only place for government interference is in matters concerning the general public health, the control of communicable diseases, the care of the tuberculous, of the chronically ill, of sufferers from nervous and mental diseases, of war veterans and of the indigent who cannot employ their own physicians. In other words, organized medicine says "socialization" shall go no farther than it already has, and organized labor says it shall. There the matter now stands. Obviously one's attitude toward this question will depend upon one's social philosophy, upon one's conception of the function of government, upon one's interpretation of the word "compulsory." It is interesting to note that those on whom the compulsion would fall are the least outraged by the idea of it. Many doctors feel that their freedom would be seriously jeopardized and their status diminished, and that medical care would deteriorate.

It is not my intention here to cast a ballot. I am not appalled by the social implications of the bill. I doubt the wisdom, however, of instituting so far reaching a reform by an act of Congress when we are as yet so inexperienced in the administration of medical care on a large scale. I should favor further experimentation with different methods of payment for services and the acquisition of more experience. We are greatly in need of intelligent leadership in this field and of codifying the facts that we are accumulating.

The adoption, with perhaps some modifications, of a plan such as Mayor LaGuardia has promulgated for New York City seems to me a step in the right direction. He has set up a nonprofit corporation under the laws of the State of New York. It is governed by a board of directors composed of representative laymen and physicians. Membership in the plan will be open to all who live or work within the city of New York. It will be subscribed to by groups, and the benefits will be available to everyone who earns up to five thousand dollars a year. The plan will cover "normal as well as catastrophic illness." It will include home, office and hospital care, specialist service, all diagnostic procedures, surgical operations, maternity care, preventive examinations and visiting-nurse service. The total charge will be approximately 4 per cent of the employees' wages, at least half to be paid by the employer and the balance by the employee. All qualified physicians will be invited to participate, so that the patient will have the widest possible choice of doctor. The physicians' salaries, it is claimed, would range from six thousand to fifteen thousand and up to twenty thousand dollars for the key men.

Although this plan is still on paper and many of its actuarial and operating details have not been worked out, it would seem to me but open-mindedness to support it in principle as a local experiment in the right direction and yet as not involving us in a sudden reform on a nation-wide scale, with administrative and other difficulties greater than we are perhaps yet ready to handle.

Whatever the future may bring in the way of the socialization of medical service, I can see no escape from the immediate disbursement of public funds for the construction of health centers. A minimum standard of hospital beds and diagnostic facilities should be set up for all communities. Where state funds are insufficient they should be supplemented by grants-in-aid from the federal government.

In this connection I should mention a plan outlined by Dr. Thomas Parran, the Surgeon General of the United States Public Health Service, in which he recommends the provision for 417,000 hospital beds and the establishment of twenty-four hundred health centers and subcenters at a cost of nearly two billion dollars. This plan does not include the needs of veterans. To his proposal should be added the establishment of mental-hygiene clinics as well. There is nothing in such a plan that need interfere with the private practice of medicine. Doctors could serve in such centers on a part-time contract basis. It would extend their usefulness and give them a backlog of financial security. They could, moreover, maintain the close personal relationship with their patients which as I have insisted and will insist again is indispensable to good medical care.

CHAPTER XVIII

Past, Present and Future

IT IS only a few years since doctors came out from behind the ambush of their beards; not so many since they laid aside their frock coats and toppers, their peaked Merlin caps and robes, their priest's vestments, their barber's aprons, their horrendous masks and drums. Today it is only taxi drivers who recognize us by the cut of our jibs. We move among laymen, stamped by no hallmarks, followed by no wake of disinfectant. No longer are we extolled as the flower of society, or ridiculed as quacks and charlatans. We are pretty much accepted for what we are—human beings with human frailties, possessing certain expert knowledge of which society has need. If we have sensitivities and mores of our own they are, in the main, looked upon indulgently as harmless vestiges.

We have, in truth, helped to unfrock ourselves. As we have forfeited our "props" and even our bedside manner, so, at the same time, have we tried to share our knowledge with others. It is now no uncommon experience for a doctor to read of an important medical discovery in the columns of his morning paper, or to learn about the use of some new drug from a "detail man" representing one of the big pharmaceutical houses. How different this from the day when we were the sole possessors of an esoteric cult, from the day when we were elite among the literati, when our title implied that we were eminently learned men and not chiropodists or chiropractors.

With the growth and dissemination of knowledge, both our

magic and our stature have diminished. But we can take comfort in solid achievement. For you who have nostalgic longings for the good old days, it is well to remember that all your swaggering and duels and brocades and nut-brown ale would probably not have carried you beyond your fortieth year, which represented then a normal expectancy of life. It is worth bearing in mind that in the last fourteen years alone the death rate from appendicitis has been reduced from 14 to 5 per 100,000, or about 60 per cent, even at a time when this illness appeared to be on the increase. This extraordinary fact can be attributed to education of the profession and of the public, and primarily to earlier diagnosis and treatment and to less frequent use of laxatives in the presence of abdominal pain.

In many respects, so it seems to me, the doctor's job is changing. He is becoming more of a teacher—in conformity with the archaic meaning of the title—and less of the wizard who compounds the serpent's wisdom and the dove's harmlessness. He is less engaged than once he was with the exorcism of evil spirits and more with the prevention of illness and with efforts to restore deranged bodily and mental functions. He is sharply aware of his own ignorance, in the face of many unsolved mysteries. And he accepts, with the late Mr. Justice Holmes, the dictum that "to live is to function." He is a mechanic—a serviceman, a repairman who instructs others in maintenance and upkeep. It is not for him to ask whether the machine is worth saving or whether its usages are noble ones. He knows something of what Thomas Huxley called "the rules of the game"—a nice Anglicism for the Laws of Nature—which govern not merely things and their forces but men and their ways as well. These the doctor attempts to impart to others less instructed than himself. "Knowledge goes to the help of Everyman." As he sees humankind in its nakedness, in its fear and weakness, in its suffering and despair, he is forced into a uniquely personal relationship. He is the harbinger of birth and often death's mighty messenger—Death, to whom

Everyman says: "Thou comest when I have thee least in mind."

His lineage is an ancient one, his task formidable. Stemming from medicine man and witch doctor, his face is now set against superstition, magic and black art, and yet he is inexorably caught up in the ignorance and bigotry of his own times. Although he began as a simple conjurer he gradually assumed the character of tribal chief and king. He became a man-god, a human being endowed with divine or supernatural powers.

In the evolution of primitive societies he constituted the oldest artificial or professional class. But the profession of exorcist has never been safe from intruders. There are always upstarts and outsiders who lay claim to healing powers—quacks, wonder workers, nature healers, patent-medicine vendors and kings. (You will recall that the young Samuel Johnson was taken before Queen Anne to be cured of scrofula.)

Among the Flathead Indians of Oregon, according to Frazer, when a man had lost his soul, he was closed up in a lodge in total darkness, after a night of dancing and singing. The medicine man, with a bunch of feathers in his hand, would brush in the lost souls through a hole in the roof of the lodge, having first carefully sorted out the appropriate one in the form of a bit of bone or a splinter of wood. He then placed this on its owner's head and with incantations patted it until it descended into the heart, and the soul returned to its proper resting place.

Now let us eavesdrop for a moment—not at the door of an Indian lodge but at a modern medicine man's office.

"Doctor, I don't know what's the matter with me. I don't feel like myself at all. The bottom's dropped out of everything. I am irritable and nasty and fly off the handle at the slightest provocation. And my mind doesn't seem to be working right. That's the worst of it. I forget everything. I can't concentrate on my work. I'm in a perfect fog. There is a wall between me and everything. I don't know who I am any more. I seem to have lost myself. I tried going to a dance last night and even getting a bit tight but it didn't do any good. I do hope you'll be able to help me. I'm sorry about the tears. Have you a bit of Kleenex? I don't usually do this sort of thing. I thought perhaps one or two talks with you would fix me up."

"Madam, I fear you have lost your soul. Just wait a minute while I take the elevator to the roof and drill a hole in it. I'll use the hearth brush and this ivory paper cutter. I'll return your soul to you. You'll soon be yourself again."

Or: "You are suffering from a retarded depression with features of agitation. It is possible that there are certain hereditary factors present, but about them we can do nothing. I am inclined to the view that psychoneurotic elements predominate. Just what the precipitating cause of your illness is, or its dynamics, I can't say without further study. I assume there is something in your present life situation that is disturbing you. There is a suicidal risk. I should prefer . . ."

"For God's sake, man, shut up. I'm not interested in science. I want to get well! Use your old feathers and splinters of bone—anything rather than this!"

In medicine's struggle with ignorance and superstition, magic gives way to religion and religion to the method of science. But always the cry from the afflicted is the same. "Help us! Heal us! Cure us! Our suffering is greater than we can bear." And the doctor is forced into the role of god-man: of Imhotep who through sacrifices restores the waters to the parched valley of the Nile, to whom the sick repair for cures; or again of Aesculapius migrating from his deep subterranean cleft in Thessaly, with his companion the Serpent, to the island of Cos, where altars were established in his honor; or even of a Christlike figure who says: "Come unto me, all ye that labor and are heavy laden."

And what do we doctors do with this archetype that is thrust upon us? We say: "If you don't mind, I will give you an injection of liver extract and vitamin B complex. That ought to help your anemia and pep you up." But supposing it does help the anemia and does not pep you up. After all, you don't complain of anemia. You complain of feeling like hell, of being all washed out. "Please, Mr. Doctor, make me well, wave a wand, do anything. I'm not interested in your science. All I want is something that works for me. Can't you understand?"

But we have to stick to our scientific guns. We shall be nonetheless scientific, and may, indeed, remain more so if we recognize and understand the constant push and pull to force us back into the role of magician, exorcist and miracle worker.

When one reflects that Greek civilization, which gave us the scientific method in medicine, was shot through with exotic religions, with belief in demonic possession, with sacrificial rites to appease angry spirits, it is indeed to their glory and to our good that they produced *physicians* who were naturalists. These Greek physicians were the first to look upon disease as phenomena of nature—to be observed, to be studied and to be recorded. They have left us, in the writings of Hippocrates and his pupils, besides the famous Oath and Precepts, numerous case reports that testify to their extraordinary powers of observation and of inductive logic.

The wife of Delearces who dwelt on the island of Thasos was seized with an acute and shivering fever. She wrapped herself in her bedclothes, was silent, fumbling, sleepless, laughed and cried and talked incoherently. On the fourteenth day of illness her breathing was "rare, large-spaced, and again hurried." (We call it Cheyne-Stokes breathing, after two Dublin physicians of the early nineteenth century. A patient of mine once referred to it as "changed-stroke" breathing, which actually describes it pretty well.) On the twentieth day she became composed and voiceless and the next day she died.

Only a very young doctor would fail to recognize this from his experience as a classical description of a typhoidal state. You will not think it ghoulish of me if I tell you that the description fills me with delight and wonder at its beauty and simplicity and accuracy, its succinctness, its dispassionate objectivity. I should not expect Delearces of Thasos, whose poor wife lay dying in this miserable state, to share my feelings. It would be hard for him to understand that inductive scientific reasoning would offer her a better chance for recovery than the sacrificial blood of a kid spilled at an altar, libations poured on the earth or a votive lamp lighted in a temple. How better can we express the ethos of good medicine than in one of the Precepts of Hippocrates: "Where the love of Man is, there also is love of the Arts"?

Grecian tablets and vase paintings show us that they cupped and bled, that they reduced dislocated shoulders and jaws. There is extant from about 490 B.C. a drinking cup bearing a painting in which Achilles is represented as bandaging the injured left upper arm of Patroclus. This was the medicine and surgery practiced in the schools at Cnidus and at Cos.

But there was also temple medicine where priests were trained in the mysteries of their cult, which they handed on from generation to generation. Exercises, baths and inunctions were used as they are today for the care of chronic diseases, and purification rituals, dream interpretation and hypnotic states were employed for the treatment of sterility and of those possessed by demons or on whom the gods had frowned.

Later, in the Middle Ages, the pagan gods were replaced by saints. Sufferers from an epidemic dancing mania which prevailed among the inhabitants of some parts of Germany frequented the chapels of St. Vitus who was believed to possess the power of curing them and whose name is now attached to the disease that we call chorea.

The histories of medicine and Christianity are closely linked, forever repeating the dramatic struggle between the rational and irrational. In the second century A.D., Christian students were excommunicated for devoting their time to the study of Galen; in the twelfth century, Benedictine friars were forbidden the study of medicine. In time, however, monastic medicine came into being and the motive of charity, as exemplified by St. Francis of Assisi, put its lasting stamp upon the practice of the healing arts, as did the motive of Christian brotherhood set the stage for latter-day social-security legislation.

What emerges from all this has been sketched with great understanding and perceptiveness by my friend Dr. Alfred Cohn, of the Rockefeller Institute for Medical Research, who says: "There has always been temple medicine—there has always been rational medicine. They have always existed side by side, they exist side by side now."

Doctors as a class are hero-worshipers. In medical history certain figures loom above their fellows because of their intellectual daring—their ability to stand alone in the very storm center of ignorance and superstition. It was Vesalius (1514–1564) who first dared perform dissections on the human body and described its anatomy; it was Harvey (1578–1657) who dared experiment and prove that the blood circulated through the arteries; it was Pasteur (1822–1895), a chemist, not a doctor of medicine, who dared propound the germ theory of disease and dispel the myth of spontaneous generation.

In addition to these great revolutionaries of science there are some few who by reason of their trenchant courage and intolerance of cant and obscurantism stand out above their generation. Foremost among these is Paracelsus (1493–1541), he of the resounding name of Philippus Aureolus Theophrastus Bombastus von Hohenheim. In some respects he was the first modern physician because he dared speak a language that others could understand (i.e., his native tongue), because he dared strip away professional pretense, because he dared to doubt and to investigate and because he recognized that (in his own words) "he who wants to know man must look upon him as a whole."

And in our own day it was Freud (1856–1941) who made himself despised among men by *looking where others dared not look*—into human passions and emotions which he regarded as natural phenomena to be observed and described, and not as the awful works of Beelzebub. He was, therefore, a marked man both for his insight into the unknown and for his infinite resolution in telling unpalatable truths. He brought reason to bear upon unreason, and in this, more than it might appear, he joined the ranks of the great scientific revolutionaries.

It is true that his followers have been forced into a kind of isolated group and have been accused by the uninformed of practicing a kind of temple medicine, pursuing a strange and costly ritual of exorcism. But it is a happy augury that the medicine of the temples and the medicine of the schools are again meeting, as they must always meet, with the wider application of the methods of science. No one will any longer deny that the work of this genius, and some of his followers, has brought light where there was darkness and has illuminated many a shadowy corner in the vast rooms of the unknown. Not only into the workings of the mind but of the body as well have we gained new insights.

The exigent demands of Selective Service, of induction, of the theaters of operation have brought psychiatry into the open. And the enormous potential for mental illness in the community has been recognized, as has the inseparable connection between anxiety and emotional conflict with symptoms of physical disability.

It is true that our knowledge is still insufficient, that our language is often gibberish, that we theorize beyond proven data. But we cannot wait for the millennium of perfect scientific comprehension before we begin to act. There is a challenge ahead of us that must be met: millions of crippled and shattered and homeless people, dislocated lives torn by unexpended hatreds and by intolerable frustrations, men and women crying as did Job: "My purposes are broken off, even the thoughts of my heart."

We must have more doctors trained in both medicine and psychiatry. Normally, we turn out about five thousand new M.D.'s annually. There are not more than some four thousand qualified psychiatrists in the United States. A large number of these work in mental hospitals and are not available to sufferers from common, though often extremely crippling, neurotic complaints. It has been estimated that there are three to five million noninstitutionalized psychiatric cases in the country. Perhaps 2 per cent or more of the population in peacetime suffer from disorders of personality severe enough to require treatment. This does not count the run-of-the-mill medical and surgical patients in the care of clinics and private doctors of whom some 50 per cent suffer from disturbances intimately connected with their emotional lives.

In Stanley Cobb's *Borderlands of Psychiatry* the picture of psychiatry in the United States in 1943 is admirably presented in diagram. Dr. Henry B. Richardson, that keen, cracker-barrel philosopher, so alive to these problems, who has recently published a valuable book with the arresting title *Patients Have Families,* once made the comment that when a clinic record reaches a certain thickness, a certain weight, the patient is usually referred for a psychiatric consultation.

Psychotherapy is lengthy and correspondingly expensive. Although the lessons learned from the war and the new techniques such as electric shock may shorten it in some selected cases, it is probable that for some years to come the principal tool will continue to be the personal interview—a time-consuming process. As yet it has not proved feasible to include this form of treatment in any prepayment health-insurance plan. The result is that we doctors are put to it to find a proper disposition for many of our cases, not only because they cannot afford to pay for treatment, but also because there simply are not enough trained men and women to take care of them. The need for more of them is pressing and obvious.

With the growth of industrial medicine and now of industrial psychiatry the time is ripe for a creative step forward. Labor and capital should combine in a disinterested project to study some of their mutual problems: absenteeism, placement, discontent, fatigue, efficiency of production, the psychological background of strikes. They could absorb their excess profits by setting up research institutes and clinics for the study and treatment of their personnel problems. It would repay them both before long.

There is almost no department of human behavior that does not fall into the province of the psychiatrist's interests: the relationship of child to parent, of men and women to each other, of individuals to groups and to society, delinquency, criminal behavior, racial hatreds and the treatment of minorities, the relationship of communities to each other, and finally even of nation to nation. As the sociologist is becoming more aware of dynamic psychology, so is the psychiatrist becoming more sociological in his thinking. Our laws are made by lawyers and our foreign policy by statesmen, diplomatists, journalists and financiers. I am so bold as to think that in this great and hazardous game of chess the psychiatrist will have something of importance to contribute to the wise move.

Throughout this book one can hear again and again two familiar antiphonal themes: the one and the many; the man and the machine. How can we safeguard the person from the mechanical contraptions we have devised to help him? If we release creative powers in him, can he use them for good beyond the drudgery of meager subsistence? Can we give to the many what now we give only to the few? Will we at last, without hypocrisy, with earnestness and justice, address ourselves to the common problems of the common man?

It has not been my intention to box the compass of medicine. Of its present we know something, of its past we know a little. We can only guess at its future. Though it is one of our daily tasks to prophesy, prognosis in medical practice is, after all, based on experience. To predict the future developments of medicine as a discipline and an art is beyond my powers. In any case I should not care to pose as a prophet. But we may be permitted our visions. Perhaps I have encompassed too much in my conception of medicine. I believe that nothing human is alien to it and that the most proper study of man is man.

Like many books this one is, I suppose, an apologia and a credo. In the accepted American tradition it should have a happy ending. William James, to whom I owe so much for the climate of my opinions, called himself a meliorist. Perhaps the world will be a better place some day, but it will be better not only for a television set in every home and for the new use of plastics. It will be better when man looks more deeply into himself and accepts responsibility for the bad as well as the good that is in him, using this crude material to mold himself and to shape and reshape his destiny.

It is part of the physician's task to contribute to this high enterprise. There are many obstacles on the way. Our patients are often skeptical. They demand miracles of us. They limit our moves by making pawns of us—or kings—when we should range freely as knights. Like other men we have to struggle for our living and do battle for our professional standards and for the scientific truth. These we fight for gladly. It is indeed a poor heart that never rejoices.

Bibliography

THE AUTHOR wishes to acknowledge his indebtedness to all those whose works he has consulted and to the publishers who have granted him permission for the use of quotations. Their names are accompanied by an asterisk.

FRONTISPIECE *Hippocrates' Oath*, translation by W. H. S. Jones, Loeb Classical Library, vol. I, Harvard University Press,* Cambridge, 1923, p. 299.

PAGE	LINE	
		Chapter I
22	10	Flexner, Simon, and Flexner, James Thomas, *William Henry Welch and the Heroic Age of American Medicine*, Viking Press,* New York, 1941.
23	3	James, Henry, *Charles W. Eliot, President of Harvard University, 1869–1909*, vol. I, Houghton Mifflin Co.,* Boston and New York, 1930, p. 289.
	14	*Ibid.*, p. 286.
		Chapter II
26	16	*American Medical Directory*, 17th edition, 1942.
32	16	Hartman, Franz, *Paracelsus*, 4th edition, Macoy and Masonic Supply Co.,* New York, 1923, p. 210.
	20	*Ibid.*, p. 205.
		Chapter III
40	31	*Ibid.*, pp. 203–204.
42	28	Sigerist, Henry E., *The Great Doctors*, translated by Eden and Cedar Paul, W. W. Norton and Co.,* New York, 1939, p. 37.
		Chapter IV
51	11	Peabody, Francis W., *The Care of the Patient*, Harvard University Press, Cambridge, 1927, p. 48.
		Chapter V
55	14	Rado, Sandor, "The Relationship of Patient to Therapist," *American Journal of Orthopsychiatry*, vol. XII, No. 3, 1942, p. 542.
57	9	Freud, Sigmund, *Collected Papers*, vol. II, Hogarth Press,* London, 1924, pp. 315–316.
60	3	Jones, Ernest, "The Concept of a Normal Mind," *International Journal of Psychoanalysis*, vol. XXIII, Part I, 1942, p. 7.
		Chapter VI
82	28	Henderson, D. K., and Gillespie, R. D., *A Textbook of Psychiatry*, 6th edition, Oxford University Press,* New York, 1944, p. 39.
	30	*Ibid.*, p. 32.
		Chapter VII
95	2	Housman, A. E., *Collected Poems*, Henry Holt and Co.,* New York, 1940, p. 232.

PAGE	LINE	
	12	Raphael, Alice, *Faust*, a translation, Jonathan Cape and Harrison Smith,* New York, 1930, p. 53.
96	23	Blitzstein, Mark, "Joe's Birthday Song," from *No for an Answer*, sung by Paul Robeson.

Chapter VIII

97	8	Jowett, B., *Dialogues of Plato*, vol. I, 3rd edition, Oxford University Press,* 1892, p. 13.
98	5	White, E. B., *Quo Vadimus*, Harper and Brothers,* New York, 1939, pp. 148–149.
104	26	Shakespeare, William, *Hamlet*, Act I, Sc. 4.
105	21	Darwin, Charles, *The Expression of the Emotions in Man and Animals*, D. Appleton and Co., New York, 1899, pp. 237–240.
106	8	Shakespeare, William, *King Henry V*, Act III, Sc. 1.
107	8	Cannon, Walter B., *Bodily Changes in Pain, Hunger, Fear and Rage. An Account of Recent Researches into the Function of Emotional Excitement*, D. Appleton and Co., New York and London, 1915. This book is out of print. It is soon to be reissued by W. W. Norton and Co.

Chapter IX

111	27	Alexander, Franz, "The Influence of Psychogenic Factors upon Gastrointestinal Disturbances, a Symposium," *Psychoanalytic Quarterly*, vol. III, No. 4, 1934, pp. 518–519.
113	18	Beaumont, William, *Experiments and Observations on the Gastric Juice and the Physiology of Digestion*, reprinted, Boston, 1929, pp. x-xiii.
116	10	Wolff, Harold G., and Wolf, Stewart, "Studies on a Subject with a Large Gastric Fistula: Changes in the Function of the Stomach in Association with Varying Emotional States," *Transactions Association, American Physicians*, vol. LVII, 1942, p. 115.
		Wolf, Stewart, and Wolff, H. G., *Human Gastric Function: An Experimental Study of a Man and His Stomach*, Oxford University Press, London, New York and Toronto, 1943.

Chapter X

124	6	Dana, Charles L., "The Story of a Great Consultation. Jerome Cardan Goes to Edinburgh," *Annals of Medical History*, vol. III, 1921, p. 122.
126	30	French, Thomas M., and Alexander, Franz, "Psychogenic Factors in Bronchial Asthma," *Psychosomatic Medicine*, Part I, Monograph IV, 1941, p. 43.

Chapter XI

133	21	Hales, Stephen, *Haemastatics*, vol. II, London, 1733, pp. 1–2.
139	26	Binger, C. A. L., Ackerman, N. W., Cohn, A. E., Schroeder, H. A., and Steele, J. M., "Personality in Arterial Hypertension," *Psychosomatic Medicine*, Monograph VIII (second series), 1945.
144	4	Hill, Lewis B., "A Psychoanalytic Observation on Essential Hypertension," *Psychoanalytic Review*, vol. XXII, 1935, pp. 60, 62, 63.

Chapter XII

148	17	Osler, William, *The Principles and Practice of Medicine*, 2nd edition, D. Appleton and Co.,* New York, 1897.

PAGE	LINE	
	20	*The Principles and Practice of Medicine,* 15th edition, by Henry A. Christian, Appleton-Century Co.,* New York, 1944.
149	4	MacDermot, H. E., "Osler's Textbook of Medicine," *McGill News,* Vol. XII, No. 4, 1931, p. 27.
	18	Flexner, Simon, and Flexner, James Thomas, *William Henry Welch and the Heroic Age of American Medicine,* op. cit.
152	23	Withering, William, *An Account of the Foxglove, and Some of Its Medical Uses; with Practical Remarks on Dropsy, and Other Diseases,* Burmingham, 1785.

Chapter XIII

156	2	Carr, James G., "Eleven Editions of Osler," *Northwestern University Bulletin,** vol. XXXIV, No. 31, 1934.
158	23	Osler, William, *The Principles and Practice of Medicine,* 8th edition, D. Appleton and Co.,* New York and London, 1912, p. 231.
159	28	*Ibid.*, 2nd edition, 1897, pp. 179–180.
160	29	*Ibid.*, pp. 156–157.
163	18	Hamilton, Alice, *Exploring the Dangerous Trades,* Little, Brown and Co., Boston, 1943.
	28	Osler, William, *op. cit.*, 2nd edition, p. 1060.
166	10	*Ibid.*, p. 700.
	29	Rous, Peyton, *The Modern Dance of Death,* the Linacre Lecture, Cambridge University Press, Macmillan Co.,* New York, 1929, p. 47.
170	2	Osler, William, *op. cit.*, 1st edition, D. Appleton and Co.,* New York, 1892, p. 412.
	10	Osler, William, *op. cit.*, 2nd edition, p. 442.

Chapter XIV

172	18	*Convalescent Care,* Committee on Public Health Relations, New York Academy of Medicine, New York, 1940.
174	1	Becker, Carl L., *The Heavenly City of the Eighteenth-Century Philosophers,* Yale University Press,* New Haven, 1932, p. 29.
176	33	Rennie, Thomas A. C., Director, Division of Rehabilitation, National Committee of Mental Hygiene. Unpublished report.
180	15	Boas, Ernst P., *The Unseen Plague—Chronic Disease,* J. J. Augustin,* New York, 1940, p. 4.
	25	*Ibid.*, p. 13.
181	6	Gregg, Alan, "The Matrix of Medicine," *Clinical Bulletin of the School of Medicine of Western Reserve University and Its Associated Hospitals,* vol. VIII, No. 1, January, 1944, p. 7.

Chapter XV

185	21	I am indebted to Dr. George Draper for the French quotation.

Chapter XVII

211	9	I am indebted to Dr. Henry E. Sigerist for these facts, as given in a lecture before the New York Academy of Medicine.
212	13	Reed, Louis S., *The Ability to Pay for Medical Care,* Publications of the Committee on the Costs of Medical Care: No. 25, University of Chicago Press, Chicago, 1933.
	19–23	Leven, Maurice, Moulton, Harold G., and Warburton, Carl, *Amer-*

PAGE LINE

ica's Capacity to Consume, Institute of Economics of the Brookings Institution, Washington, D. C., Publication No. 56, 1934, p. 54.

19–23 *Consumers' Incomes in the United States: Their Distribution in 1935–36,* National Resources Committee, United States Government Printing Office, Washington, 1938, p. 18.

19–23 *Sales Management,* "Survey of Buying Power," April 10, 1940, p. 54.

19–23 *Civilian Spending, 1941–1942,* Office of Price Administration, Division of Research, Consumer Income and Demand Branch Publication, March 1, 1943.

213 16 Leland, R. G., "Income from Medical Practice," *Journal of the American Medical Association,* vol. XCVI, No. 20, Chicago, 1931, p. 1683.

214 17 Leland, R. G., *Distribution of Physicians in the United States,* Bureau of Medical Economics, American Medical Association, Chicago (revised May, 1936).

215 6 *Wartime Health and Education,* hearings before a subcommittee of the Committee on Education and Labor, United States Senate, 78th Congress, Part 5, United States Government Printing Office, Washington, 1944.

218 34 Avnet, Helen Hershfield, *Voluntary Medical Insurance in the United States: Major Trends and Current Problems,* Medical Administration Service, Inc., New York, 1944.

220 7 Mannix, John R. "Voluntary Non-Profit Prepayment for Health Care," *Journal of the American Medical Association,* vol. CXXIV, No. 9, 1944, p. 571.

Chapter XVIII

227 16 Frazer, Sir James George, *The Golden Bough,* Macmillan Co., New York, 1926, p. 187.

229 10 Singer, Charles, *Greek Biology and Greek Medicine,* Oxford University Press, American Branch, 1922.

231 6 Cohn, Alfred E., "Changes in Public Attitudes toward Medicine: Historical Aspects," *Bulletin of the History of Medicine,* vol. XI, No. 1, 1942, p. 31.

233 12 Cobb, Stanley, *Borderlands of Psychiatry,* Harvard University Press, Cambridge, 1943.

14 Richardson, Henry B., *Patients Have Families,* Commonwealth Fund, New York, 1944.

Index

For Product Safety Concerns and Information please contact our EU representative GPSR@taylorandfrancis.com Taylor & Francis Verlag GmbH, Kaufingerstraße 24, 80331 München, Germany